The Simple
And
Natural Way

*...to Perfect Weight, Radiant Health
and Transformed Life*

SHAILAJA PRASHANT KEDARI

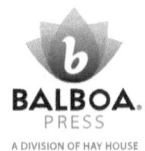

BALBOA.
PRESS

A DIVISION OF HAY HOUSE

Balboa Press books may be ordered through booksellers or by contacting:

Balboa Press
A Division of Hay House
1663 Liberty Drive
Bloomington, IN 47403
www.balboapress.com
1-(877) 407-4847

ISBN: 978-1-4525-6284-1 (sc)
ISBN: 978-1-4525-6285-8 (e)

Because of the dynamic nature of the Internet, any web addresses or links contained in this book may have changed since publication and may no longer be valid. The views expressed in this work are solely those of the author and do not necessarily reflect the views of the publisher, and the publisher hereby disclaims any responsibility for them.

The author of this book does not dispense medical advice or prescribe the use of any technique as a form of treatment for physical, emotional, or medical problems without the advice of a physician, either directly or indirectly. The intent of the author is only to offer information of a general nature to help you in your quest for emotional and spiritual well-being. In the event you use any of the information in this book for yourself, which is your constitutional right, the author and the publisher assume no responsibility for your actions.

Any people depicted in stock imagery provided by Thinkstock are models, and such images are being used for illustrative purposes only.
Certain stock imagery © Thinkstock.

Printed in the United States of America

Balboa Press rev. date: 11/12/2012

Contents

To Horace Fletcher (1849–1919), To my loved ones,
To Nature, To God

What This Book is About

There is this very simple and natural way to **radiant health**. It is a path very commonly known but not frequently travelled. It is very effective and delivers what it promises. It's the Natures answer to all the health related questions. This natural remedy promises vigor and increased stamina. It promises to keep your immune system at its protective best, not letting in any seasonal, occasional or routine viruses of any shape or form. It promises to take you to the peak of your strength and endurance, a level you could probably never have imagined was possible for you to achieve. **Perfect weight** i.e. weight loss if you are overweight and weight gain if you are underweight is an essential byproduct of this process. It promises to help quit smoking and other addictions too eventually–sooner than later. It reaches out further and touches every aspect of your being–the way you think, talk, walk, breathe, and live your life! It **transforms your life!**

It's not a product or a service you need to purchase. It's not something you need to eat or drink in addition to your usual diet. You don't need to be spending an extra penny on any program, routine or counseling. Rather you would be saving quite some money to say the least. You don't have to be taking time out to do 10 different things. You don't have to force yourself to give up anything you love. There will be noticeable changes within a short period of time if you practice it sincerely, in the way you eat, drink, live your life, but it will be a natural, pleasant transition with very little or no resistance from any part of your being.

You don't have to believe that it works, give it a fair try and the results will make you a believer!

This book is about this simple, natural, commonly and widely known but sparsely practiced way of eating, the Natures way, called Fletcherism, named after Horace Fletcher (1849–1919).

Introduction

For me the results Fletcherism promised seemed too good to be true initially, until I started giving it a fair try and realized that yes, it is too good and it is very true!

A physical, mental and emotional transformation has taken place and continues to take place in my life since I started walking the path of Fletcherism. The speed with which this is occurring still amazes me as to how something so simple and natural can work this swiftly, this effectively, and this magically!

The transformation was so visible to everyone around me that before I could go out and share the reasons behind it with them, I had my family, friends, colleagues and neighbors coming up to me asking what I've been up to. Even those who did not know me or had never spoken to me but had noticed me on my way to work or at the grocery store or seen me taking a walk in the neighborhood started asking me about this. They had seen the first and physical signs of my transformation–weight loss, quick and very much apparent. So much so that my entire frame had shrunk within a very short time, head to toe. I started looking much younger, so completely different than I used to look. I was told by some that they did not recognize me at first when they saw me at a distance. Honestly, this was way over what I was expecting with Fletcherism! It made me feel very happy to be able to share my experience with and guide all those who have been coming to me for help since the past few months. And now, it gives me great pleasure to share it with you!

To summarize what I had achieved to begin with—In about 15 weeks time (end of Feb, 2012 to end of May 2012), I had lost 30 pounds of weight—head to toe. This was even when I was eating my regular food, not taking any weight loss medicine or supplement and with only moderate level of activity—walking for about 20 to 25 minutes daily. My friends would jokingly ask, "Where have you left the other half of you?" They said that had they not seen the transition, right in front of their eyes, from the "plump" and "chubby" me to the lean me, they would never have believed that something so simple can work so fast and so effectively.

For me personally, it's nothing short of a miracle because of the pace with which it works, miracle because of the meal time pleasure it gives and miracle because of state of health I am in and advancing to!

This weight loss was only an outward first sign of the shift that was occurring in my life. This was only the tip of the iceberg. I did not realize this until I started talking to those who asked, giving them tips, telling them the how, why, what of the entire process. The more I spoke about Fletcherism, the more I realized what it was all about. I realized that it is fool proof preventive health maintenance and also a successful cure to the several ailments we suffer—directly and directly connected to our intake of nourishment—food and drinks. I realized it was changing my lifelong habits—not just of eating!

What I had been practicing and continue to practice now is something everyone I speak to already knows about, theoretically. It is strange though to see that no one (including me until recently) actually thinks of giving it a fair trial. To work as per Natures design first, before deciding to torture ourselves with diet restrictions, forced workout routines, resultant resistance from mind-body and ultimate disappointments in majority of the cases.

In his book, "Fletcherism—what is it and how I became young at 60" Fletcher says: *"For five months I went on patiently observing, and I found out positively in that time that I had worked out my own salvation. I had lost upwards of sixty pounds of fat: I was feeling better in all ways than I had for twenty years. My head was clear, my body felt springy, I enjoyed walking, I had not had a single cold for five months, "that tired feeling" was gone!"*

2 + 2 always equals 4. This is how Fletcherism works, it works for everyone and the results are guaranteed. What Fletcherism did to Horace Fletcher, it is doing to me and it will do to you:

- You will enjoy more than ever, every bite of food you eat, every sip of milk, tea or juices you drink. Even the simplest piece of bread will taste so amazingly delicious, it would be so surprising and unbelievable at times! If you love food, you will love it all the more!
- You will lose weight—faster than probably you ever have in all your life so far. It will be very apparent in the first couple of months itself (I lost about 20 pounds in the first 2.5 months). And if you are underweight, you will gain weight!
- You will feel lighter in your body and your head. If physical activities like walking, jogging, exercising, climbing up the stairs, trekking tired you in the past, they will not anymore to the degree they did, and not at all eventually. You will feel like going for a walk and will not have to force yourself to do it. For me, I have started enjoying now, my erstwhile tiring and boring walks. 25 minutes of walking would usually be a drag in the past, but now I don't seem to notice how 25 minutes fly by, it feels so effortless. It feels quite springy walking around, it's like a big weight has been lifted off—head to toe.
- You may feel tempted to take the stairs, not to "do your bit" to stay healthy or save electricity, but to test your new found heath, fitness and vigor, to surprise yourself!
- The possibility of putting on excess weight will seem quite remote and the fear of falling sick will seem to be fading away. You will know that every cell of your body is getting healthier by the day and will protect itself from all the infections, viruses and germs.
- Your energy—mental, physical and at all times of the day will seem to be constantly increasing and "that tired feeling" at the end of a working day, which, if it used to be the norm, will

now be a rare occurrence. Your capacity to work will seem to have increased.

- The way you walk, talk, breathe, feel about your body, about yourself–in and out, would dramatically shift in every sense. You will feel so comforted, happy and safe knowing that you are taking care of yourself in the best possible way. You will feel so wonderfully pampered. You won't need to force yourself to eat what you don't want to or don't eat what you want to. You will not have to exercise "to stay healthy" but you will be motivated to be more active physically because a healthy body cannot be inactive.
- You will have people–family, friends, acquaintances, coming up to you to know your "secret", to know what you have been doing. You will be able to guide them, help them with their own health problems.
- Even on your fiftieth birthday, you will enjoy the strength and endurance to ride two hundred miles on your bicycle and come home feeling fine. Would you be stiff the next day? Not at all, and you will ride another fifty miles the next morning in order to test the effect of your stunt and you would find yourself ready again to ride another 200 miles. This is not wishful thinking, Horace Fletcher did this and many such stunts to prove to himself and to the world what miracles are possible with Fletcherism.
- Other aspects of your personality, your priority setting skills, your belief system about Natures laws and how they work, your knowledge and experience about the role you play in creating your life, your "compassion quotient" towards others, your ideas about the values you wish to instill into your children–everything will undergo a change. Heck! Your dreams may come true, your wishes may get fulfilled–that's what I have started to experience now.

Fletcherism can help make all this possible, it has made all this possible for Horace Fletcher and number of Fletcherites before and after him. It is making it possible for me, it will for you.

It can be a helping hand, a ray of hope to the multitude of people struggling with health, weight, strength and endurance issues. It can help you, if you wish to be helped; to live your life to the fullest possible potential of your physical body and it will also touch the non–physical one in profound ways.

About Horace Fletcher

Horace Fletcher (1849–1919), an American Health-food enthusiast, has been immortalized with his name being assigned to this practice of treating and preparing food in the mouth in a way that the food is easily digested, thoroughly assimilated and absorbed in the body, taking the body to its highest level of health, strength and endurance.

Horace Fletcher, known as "The Great Masticator" recommended chewing food at least once for every tooth or 32 times per mouthful before swallowing (our Grandmas told us too). Fletcher would chew a morsel 100 times a minute before swallowing and believed (rightly so) that this opened the flood gates of health, strength, energy, vigor and endurance, which is naturally inbuilt in each and every one of us but is just lying dormant, waiting to be unleashed. Fletcher submitted himself to various experiments on his strength and endurance in his 50s and 60s, the results of which surprised or even seemed miraculous to the doctors, physicians, the young college students and trained professional athletes.

Fletcher's books "Fletcherism—what is it and how I became young at 60" and "The New Glutton or Epicure" explain the theory and practice of Fletcherism. They record the details of various experiments conducted on Fletcher and those conducted by Fletcher on others proving the results, the effectiveness of Fletcherism. They explain how Fletcherism has changed bodies, transformed lives!

These books, the experiments, the findings, have been a source of inspiration and guidance for me. They got me started on this fascinating new way of life. Several of Fletchers notes on the subject and the findings of the experiments as written in these books have been included in here, in this book as it would be impossible to talk about Fletcherism without including these notes and experiments.

I am grateful to Horace Fletcher, all those who have aided him in his research and those who have contributed to this practice before Fletcher came on screen. They have all been the catalyst of the most important transformation in the lives of the many struggling to find the best way out of all the health related issues.

1

Fletcherism–Natures Design & Guidance

Every Creation of the Creator comes with an inbuilt natural mechanism which aids its survival and nourishment in the best possible way. Animals, birds, plants, bees, worms and every so called simpler forms of life know exactly when to eat, how to eat, what to eat and how much to eat. Let's leave aside the domesticated animals and plants for the time being where we humans seem to have an influence over their nutrition. What about wild life, the vegetation in the forest? Who prescribes a diet for them, who gives the trees and flowers the precise amount of water, rather who decides what is the exact quantity of water they need and at what times and intervals? None of us might have seen, heard or for that matter can even imagine an animal or a tree in the forest overeating and growing fat. How do they know the "When, How, What and How much" of nutrition? Does anyone outside of them decide this? Does anyone give them a diet chart to follow with a prescribed intake of proteins, vitamins, minerals, carbs etc? Is it not their natural design, the way they were created by the creator, their body and brain, that guides them to the "When, How, What and How Much" of Nourishment?

Would it be right then to assume that a more complex and higher form of creation, we humans, come without this inbuilt mechanism? No it would not be right to assume so. There is no manufacturing defect where it comes to us humans, we have been equally gifted

1

with this inbuilt mechanism. Just that we don't seem to be utilizing it to the best possible use it is capable of. It is kind of lying unutilized or underutilized and is probably rusting away because of this.

This built in mechanism, this internal guidance is available to us all the time, and it keeps sending constant signals guiding us to our own good. Would these constant signals that provide us guidance every step of our way be so complex that they need decoding by an expert? Or are they so very simple that we look straight past it or worse still ignore it even though we are aware of what it is that we are receiving?

They are very simple, very direct, very visible and physical signs. These signs are no way subtle or difficult to read so cannot be ignored unless one really decides to ignore, consciously or subconsciously. These signs direct us perfectly to observe and follow the Natures way; the essence of it is what Fletcherism is all about. It is captured in the five principles noted by Fletcher.

The five principles of Fletcherism

In "Fletcherism—What is it or how I became young at 60", Fletcher notes:

THE FIVE PRINCIPLES OF FLETCHERISM

I have now found out five things; all that there is to my discovery relative to optimum nutrition; and to the fundamental requisite of what is called Fletcherism.

First   : Wait for a true, earned appetite

Second : Select from the food available that which appeals most to appetite, and in the order called for by appetite.

Third   : Get all the good taste there is in food out of it in the mouth, and swallow only when it practically "swallows itself.""

Fourth   : *Enjoy the good taste for all it is worth, and do not allow any depressing or diverting thought to intrude upon the ceremony.*

Fifth   : *Wait; take and enjoy as much as possible what appetite approves; Nature will do the rest*

These five principles summarize all the physical aspects involved in Fletcherism and the "action" that needs to be taken by an individual based on the signs and guidance received from within. These principles specify, in no uncertain terms, "When, How, What and How much to eat". It is not a dietary prescription given by Fletcher or any of the Doctors or Physicians. Fletcherism does not prescribe a standard quantity, quality, time or frequency of meals. It does not prescribe what type of food has to be eaten and what type not to be eaten. This is what increases the "Acceptance Quotient" of Fletcherism with Foodies as well. Every aspect of Fletcherism is entirely left upon the individual to decide for himself, for herself, based on his or her unique "Default Factory settings", his own internal guidance, her own inner voice and signs, which by the way are very physical signs and so not very difficult to read.

When, How, What and How much to eat

When to eat

"Eat when you are Hungry and Good" says Fletcher. These are two very physical and apparent signs. We would know when we are Hungry and we would know when we are good.

Hunger is the body's natural built in mechanism saying "I am ready for food". After sufficient activity when the body has used up the energy generated from the nutrition that was fed to it, it expresses its need for a refill. This need for a refill, to be able to run this magnificent, powerful machine, is expressed in the form of Hunger or a "Natural Appetite" as Fletcher puts it.

Hunger as I and most of us have known is that "not very pleasant" feeling in the stomach. The feeling of emptiness, the vacuum created in there which seems to suck up our entire being into it at times, the times when we think we are really very hungry and starving. This feeling is no way a pleasant and "looking forward to and excited about eating" feeling. It is so urgent! Some of us have this headache if we remain hungry for a longer period of time. We experience that weakness of sorts in our head and body. There is this urgency to eat, as if you have to eat first else you cannot concentrate on the work at hand or get anything done. It may not be this severe for everyone all the time, but almost everyone might have experienced these unpleasant feelings and called it hunger at least sometimes.

On this Fletcher says: *"Normal Appetite is Nature's means of indicating her fuel and repair requirements for the Mind Power-Plant.*

Study Normal Appetite and heed its invitation. It prescribes wisely. Its mark of distinction, to differentiate it from False Appetite is "watering of the mouth" for some particular thing.

False Appetite is an indefinite craving for something, anything! To smother disagreeable sensations and frequently is expressed by the symptom of "faintness" or "All-gone-ness"

The "Unpleasant Hunger" is not the "Natural Hunger". All these symptoms of the unpleasant hunger are bodies healing mechanism working to correct the internal digestive disorders, to "clean the house", to pave the way for the Natural Hunger to make its appearance. True earned appetite or hunger does not show up till these symptoms have disappeared. Eventually once you become a Fletcherite, these symptoms will cease to be generated since the house will always be clean.

Natural Hunger or Natural Appetite is that pleasant feeling in the mouth evidenced by an increase in secretion of saliva, not forcefully created by smelling, tasting or imagining food, but produced simply and naturally because you are hungry. It is that pleasant feeling of the body preparing itself to receive food, the major source of its nourishment and nutrition, the anticipation of incoming life giving source that keeps us alive.

When the body has been prepared for receiving the food, all the digestive juices ready to pamper the incoming food and every cell of the body ready to absorb the nutrition, that's when a very physical sign is sent to our salivary glands, to our taste buds, that's when the pleasant anticipation begins, the taste buds start tingling, the mouth starts watering. There is no urgency here, it is only pleasant and exciting, and it is Natural Hunger.

It seems only logical that if thirst is something we feel in our mouth, on our tongue and not in our stomach, hunger as well is felt in the mouth. Thirst is the body's need for water conveyed to the mouth in the form of dryness in the mouth. When we drink and the body has received enough water, the satisfaction of water requirement is again communicated to the mouth and it's no longer dry. So why should hunger be any different? When the body needs food, it sends this sign to that part of the body through which food will enter, the mouth and the signal is the secretion of saliva, the tingling of the taste buds, the Natural Hunger.

This sign though quite obvious and strong, gets lost in the overriding feeling in the stomach, the "so called" hunger. To let the natural hunger resurface, Fletcher advises those who can, to skip a meal or two if possible, to see the urgency die down, to see the unpleasant hunger disappear, and to really understand what true hunger is.

Why is being in a good mood while eating important? All of us know what stress, anxiety, bad mood, fear, anger does to the body. It releases chemicals in the body which are nothing short of poison, only that it's a slow poison. We don't die immediately but eventually it takes the toll on our health and well being. It's advisable to be in a good mood always though, every moment of our life, if not, at least when eating!

Unpleasant thoughts interfere with the natural, normal functioning of our digestive system. For example; you can see for yourself that bad mood stops or slows down the secretion of saliva. Now this is a very physical sign which we can notice but we can only imagine or maybe even not imagine what's happening inside the body, to the other digestive juices, to the entire digestion, distribution and assimilation process. If you are having your dinner over an argument at the table, the food loses its charm, the body is not able to process the food and derive nutrition from it naturally and effortlessly and it has to bear the additional burden of moving all the waste through the digestive track and then throwing it out. The dinner was a waste in every sense, even from a financial point of view. It would do only good in that case to keep discussions on Politics, News & Views and Current Affairs also out of the dining room and wait until we get back to our happy selves before we eat.

There is no standard time table set forth that needs following for breakfast, lunch and dinner. There are only two words, two feelings that say it all—"Hungry" and "Good". Only you would know when you feel these. If midnight is when you feel both—eat then, but Fletcherise, is what Fletcher advises.

How to eat:

The natural design of the body parts which are used in the process of eating and digestion itself speaks clearly about how they were meant to be used in the process and *how* are we to eat.

The front end of the Mouth is bigger than the rear end towards the throat, where the tongue falls back to its roots—the passage through which food flows down into the stomach by the act of swallowing. Teeth are located in the mouth. Saliva is generated in the mouth. The taste buds have been given in the mouth. So the Creator is indicating in no uncertain terms that mouth is the field designated for action. If stomach was where all these tools had been given, we would know that's where all the action should take place. But that's not the case.

When a morsel of food is put into the mouth a series of actions take place, mostly involuntary based on how we have been taught to eat. We also add our own refinements to the process and eventually it turns into a habit. The food touches the tongue, the taste buds receive the taste and there is an increase in the secretion of saliva. The jaws move, the food is moved around, center, sideways, in circles by the tongue, and the teeth start grinding the food. When this action is taking place in the mouth, the rear end of the mouth is shut tight. It's a kind of "Food Filter" (as Fletcher puts it) there which prevents accidental swallowing. Habitual swallowing if is kind of gulping down half chewed food; this Food Filter is forcefully opened to push the food in. For most of us swallowing means a voluntary gulping down of food or drinks. This again is a force of habit done unconsciously. This gulping down or voluntary swallowing is actually an unwanted intervention in the natural process.

Nature has designed this activity of eating in the most harmonic manner which includes the automatic opening of the Food filter to allow "involuntary swallowing" of the food which is ready to be swallowed. It would be very strenuous to personally keep a track of each of the activity and try to "run" it yourself. It's like trying to keep the heart beating, the blood circulating voluntarily, consciously; it's beyond our capacity to do this. Rather we are not required to do this. The inbuilt intelligence takes care of these involuntary processes. Likewise the act of eating, preparing the food for digestion and then letting it fall down involuntarily for further processing is also taken care of by the intelligence with only one bit where we are required to fulfill our responsibility, where we are required to do our duty. We are required to taste it as much as we can. Mindful tasting sets in motion the other processes in perfect synchronicity which eventually gets the food to a state where it is ready to be swallowed.

The food is ready to be swallowed when the taste buds are satisfied so that there is no more taste left to be extracted from the morsel, the teeth have finished grinding so that there is not even a smallest piece left unattended, and the saliva is completely mixed with the food breaking it down to its most digestion and nourishment friendly form. It is at this stage the food filter opens up naturally and automatically to allow this rich and nutritious mixture to flow down into the stomach, involuntarily.

It's like eating a chewing gum. We chew on it till we extract the last drop of the sugary juices, maybe chew it even then for a while but eventually, the gum is spit out. If at all the gum has been swallowed which most of us have done in our childhood, or do even now sometimes, it is accidental and not intentional. This is what needs to be done with every food we put into our mouth.

What's the point in swallowing something which still has some taste left in it? Would it not be taste gone waste? There is nothing in the stomach that can appreciate taste; it can only appreciate food thoroughly prepared for digestion. So mouth has to get every bit of taste out of the food and then pass on the "prepared" food to the stomach. They both–the tongue and the stomach get what they want–it's a complete WIN WIN!

In the habitual (and often incorrect) way of eating, when the activity of chewing is going on, the food seems to stay in the center of the mouth, on the tongue, and un-chewed food seems to be going towards the food filter to be swallowed. When Fletcherising, it becomes very apparent that Nature has given these "parking lots" in the sides of the mouth–the space between the lower set of teeth and cheek. You will notice these "parking spaces" seem to stay vacant or underutilized most of the times when adults are eating; children park the food there forever. It has been given to serve a purpose, the purpose of parking the food waiting to be chewed. The danger in not utilizing these parking spaces is that the food stays at the center of the mouth, getting partially chewed, not fully tasted yet losing its taste because of the haphazard treatment. The food, in a nutshell, becomes unmanageable and goes straight to be swallowed. These parking spaces retain the taste in the food and keep adding fresh supply of taste to the grinding and insalivation process, making it all the more enjoyable.

On this Fletcher says: *"Taste is excited by the dissolving of food in the mouth, and while it lasts a necessary process of preparation for digestion is going on.*

The juices of the mouth have the power to transform any food that excites taste into a substance suitable for the body.

Nothing that is tasteless, except water and pure protied, only by distinct invitation of appetite, should be taken into the stomach. If we swallow only the food which excites the appetite and is pleasing to the sense of taste, and swallow it only after the taste has been extracted from it, removing from the mouth the tasteless residue, complete and easy digestion will be assured and perfect health maintained."

That which the teeth cannot grind and saliva cannot liquefy, penetrate and break down, needs to be removed out of the mouth. This is because there is no other grinder as strong and natural as the teeth and no digestive juice as miraculous as the saliva anywhere else in our body. To begin with why would we want to swallow something from which all the nutrients have been extracted and where there is no scope of any further processing like for example the fibrous remains of meat, the outer shell of corn, the seeds of some fruits?

If say the fibrous remains of meat or un-chewed food is gulped down and passed on for further processing, what happens to it is this. Our helpless and toothless intestines take the aid of the scavenger bacteria in our body to break down and decompose the matter. This decomposed matter is partially passed out of the body as the digestive ash (excreta) after passing through the 20 to25 feet long intestines, utilizing our precious brain energy in the process. It is then partially absorbed into the body as unrequired fat, and rest is circulated as toxins (and not nourishment) in the blood. So impurities galore, everywhere, in every single cell of our body, only because removing the un-chewed remains may go against the table manners or worse still we are too busy to be mindful of what is passing un-chewed down the throat.

"Nature will castigate those who don't masticate"" was Fletchers war cry!

Masticating well does not mean eating slow. Fletcher, "The Great Masticator" was known to be able to chew every morsel a 100 times within a minute before it was involuntarily swallowed. This is vigorous chewing, which comes naturally, but with some practice. This vigorous jaw movement also encourages secretion of saliva. Watering of mouth does take place evidencing hunger, but when in contact with food, jaw action seems to set free a far greater flow of saliva. This logically is essential to lubricate, break down the food and prepare it for digestion. It seems Nature intended this vigorous movement of the jaw and so has designed it in a way which provides it the maximum flexibility and speed to carry out its functions.

Some may wonder why bother so much? If liquid is what does it, will not a liquid diet be a better idea? The food will be in a liquid state and so prepared for digestion! But then one important catalyst will be missing in the process, the catalyst which really prepares food for digestion. Saliva, the digestive! Liquid food gulped down is maybe a little less harmful but it still does great harm. Looking at the natural design of the body, we have been given teeth for some useful purpose; babies don't have it so it's okay to feed them liquid till their teeth have erupted.

On the subject of adults being on a liquid diet, Fletcher notes "*Liquid for adults, for anyone after the eruption of teeth, is an artificial and unnatural sustenance; something not taken into consideration when the human body was planned. Liquid food (drunk without mixing with saliva) is a sort of nutritive self-abuse, and the only way to avoid the ill effect is to give it the same chance to encounter saliva that the constituent ingredients would have had in a more solid state.*"

There could be those, especially in old age, who don't have strong teeth anymore or even strong jaws. They probably are already on a liquid or semi liquid diet. Fletcherising is not limited to solid food. So this liquid or semi liquid intake can be Fletcherised as well.

It is really amazing how Nature has taken care of every detail; it has not missed anything and has given us every perfect tool in our very own body, to make perfect use of, and to make the most of!

What to eat:

"*Whatever it is that is called by the appetite and in the order called by the appetite*", is what Fletcher says.

Out of the several options laid out on the table, whatever catches your attention first is what you eat. As Fletcher puts it, if the body needs starch in that moment, the craving will be for Potatoes or any other food rich in starch. If desserts are what the appetite calls for first instead of the starters or the main course, feel free to have them till you feel satisfied, then if you still have some hunger left, look for the next best option and so on. However it's important to note that deciding at the very beginning that "I will eat starters first, then the main course and then the desserts" will only lead to overeating. It's good to let the appetite and natural instincts take charge.

Sometimes there is this feeling of overwhelm looking at the various delicious and mouth watering variety of food laid upon the table or listed on the menu card. There is this beast within which wants to have everything and take possession of all it can lest someone finish it off before we get our hands on it. There is this urge to eat as much as possible which clouds the judgment and leads to incorrect choices. This issue of not being able to overcome the initial urge is addressed in the chapter "Fletcherism–Making it a Habit"

Even if we overcome the initial urge and think calmly, it may be difficult in the beginning to distinguish between the genuine appetite and the habitual craving. We do receive signs pulling us to something else and not what we are habituated to eat. However this sign appears to be very subtle compared to the overriding urge to eat what Habit prescribes. It does get confusing. But if we simply resolve to Fletcherise and stick to the resolve of Fletcherising no matter what it is that we are eating, even if it is that prescribed by habit, we will soon be able to receive these indications more clearly from our body. We will be able to differentiate between habitual craving and genuine appetite. It gets even better when the habitual craving completely transitions into genuine appetite and you don't have to think a second before choosing your pick. The initial worry and fear of choosing the wrong food and its resultant impact on our health disappears, leaving behind a sense of well being and satisfaction.

The shift I have experienced in my choice of foods within 15 weeks is nothing short of a miracle for me and for all those who were familiar with my erstwhile eating habits. I loved non-vegetarian food; I still love it but don't choose it over other options available. I have almost turned a vegetarian without any mental, moral or religious force pushing me towards this transition. I do have my share of desserts and comfort food. It's just that the quantity I consume is greatly reduced accompanied by an increase of meal time pleasure. This naturally happens to every Fletcherite. He does not have to force himself to give up the food he loves, she does not have to deprive herself of what she wants to eat and eat what someone says she should be eating. The change in the personal menu card is inevitable, just that you will still eat what you love and love more than ever, what you eat!

How much to eat:

"Wait; take and enjoy as much as possible what appetite approves; Nature will do the rest", says Fletcher.

Most of us have received, more often than not, a sign saying "please stop" from our overfull tummies and our tired brains. With Fletcherising we receive this sign sooner, at a more appropriate time, from a satisfied, happy tummy and a grateful brain.

How much to eat basically depends on the appetite which in turn depends on the level of activity the body is engaged in. An office goer's quantity of intake differs greatly from a wood cutters. Even for an office goer a day with higher level of physical activity will generate more appetite than the other days of inactivity. The type and quantity of food required also varies based on the climatic conditions. Cooler weather will demand more quantity and a different type of food than summer does. So there is no standard prescription on the quantity of food that needs to be consumed. This again like all other aspects of Fletcherism is to be decided by the Fletcherite under the expert guidance of Nature.

The Community of Doctors agree and Science has proven that when the pace with which food falls into the digestive track is slow, the message that one has eaten enough reaches the brain quickly and in time to avoid overeating. Rather it will be noticed as soon as one starts Fletcherising, that the quantity of food usually consumed is greatly reduced, starting from the very first time, the very first day one Fletcherises. Hence a check on overeating right away!

Much of the overeating takes place because of the habitual cravings and the quick speed of eating that some have. When food is taken in and gulped down with speed, the taste buds do not seem to be satisfied even though the stomach is getting filled up. The sense of smell too at times plays the trick but not as strong as the sense of taste does. With Fletcherising though, the taste buds are completely satisfied first since we take in all the taste we can from every single bite before sending in the food down to the stomach. There are very few among us I believe who will continue to eat when their tongue says "I don't want more".

Something very noticeable happens to our habitual cravings when we are down with a very bad cold, the kind of cold which robs us of our sense of taste and smell. Do we feel like eating anything at all? I find it difficult to believe that a person so down with cold will enjoy his meal in the usual fashion or would even think of overeating. We would eat the bare minimum to make sure we are not starving. I remember being offered my favorite desserts on couple of these "down with cold and no taste" occasions. I did not find it difficult to say no. I remember having thought to myself, "What's the point in eating that and increasing my calorie intake when I can't even enjoy the taste". My cravings suddenly disappeared and came back only when my sense of taste and smell returned. So it's the taste buds more than anything else which seem to regulate powerfully the quality and quantity of food consumed. Fletcherising keeps the taste buds satisfied and so helps avoid overeating.

On overeating Fletcher notes: *"Imposition upon the body of any excess of food or drink is one of the most dangerous and far reaching of self abuses; because whatever the body had no need of at the moment must be gotten rid of at the expense of much valuable energy taken away from brain service. Hence it is that when there is intestinal constipation, the energy reserve is lowered enormously, and even where there is no painful obstruction, the mere passage of waste through some twenty to twenty five feet of convoluted intestinal canal is a great tax upon available mental and physical power"*

The amount of hard work put in by anyone to earn a living is very little compared to the hard work that goes on within the body. Even if that's a wood cutter, a miner, a construction worker or a professional athlete, all of whom are required to exert physically. The energy expended without is tiny looking at the brain energy employed within in the process of digestion, distribution and assimilation of the food taken in. Any un-Fletcherised food passing through the Food Filter or any bite eaten after the natural appetite is satisfied drains the precious brain energy enormously. The energy when freed up can offer itself to the development of our muscles, tissues and bones and can take our physical self to its peak potential.

Most of us have been told in the childhood, and hence have become habituated to finish whatever is in the plate. We in turn pass on the same message to our little ones. The intention is good, that we do not want to be "wasting" food. If however finishing off whatever is in the plate results in overeating, it is a waste much higher in magnitude with far reaching consequences. The food if left on the plate is wasted, only the food is wasted. If it is taken in the body instead; the food is wasted, the brain energy is wasted, the quantity of toxins running in our cells, in our blood is increased, our health is wasted in a nutshell! Of course food wastage can be avoided, but by taking lesser amount on the plate in the first place, which a Fletcherite does. Eating it is not even close to avoiding wastage. It tantamounts to sabotaging ones health.

E. W. Redfield who witnessed Fletchers endurance test–a test where Fletcher, at the age of 50, rode in a day, more than 304 kilometers or 190 miles on a cycle (not today's gear driven light weight models, but the machines available in the 1900's), observed, *"…and the only thing I couldn't discover was how a man who ate so little could travel so far and seem never to get tired."* This amply proves it's not the quantity of food consumed which gives strength and endurance to the body, it is the quality. Quality doesn't mean the ingredients and the method or form in which it is cooked, the spices used, the herbs used etc.

Quality means the food that is prepared for digestion–thoroughly Fletcherised food.

A Fletcherite cannot over eat or even under eat for that matter. A Fletcherite will eat just right, not by chance, not occasionally or usually, but ALWAYS!

2

Like Wine Tasters Taste Wine

Drinks usually do not get parked in the mouth for as long as food does, reason being, it's already in a liquid form so we recon it's not important to Fletcherise.

Fletcher suggests that's not how it is, "*The first thought that will arise in the reader's mind will undoubtedly be, "What! Masticate milk, soups, wines, spirits, and other liquids; nonsense! That is impossible!"*

It is not, however, impossible, and, furthermore, it is absolutely necessary to protection against abuse of the stomach and possible disease.

The only things necessary to life that we are compelled to take into the body that do not excite the sense of taste are pure air and pure water. These are necessary to life, but are not what is called nutrition. They do not, alone, replace waste tissue. They do not challenge the sentient, Taste, and hence do not require retention in the field of taste."

Any liquid, therefore, which has a taste, needs mastication to prepare it for digestion. That's how toothless babies or little children eat their liquid food, they salivate profusely and they keep the liquid food in the mouth for a very long time. They do this even with water as if telling us, "Even this needs some mouth treatment".

In an experiment conducted on a person whose stomach was very sensitive, sensitive to an extent that there would be a mild protest–a sort of a shrug of the shoulders, as it were, when the person took milk or soup, Fletcher notes, "…*and that when the same liquids have been moved about in the mouth for the time necessary to naturally excite the Swallowing Impulse, they have passed into the stomach without the owner being conscious afterwards of their presence except by feeling of complete satisfaction*"

Mother's milk is alkaline in Nature, something which is easily digested by the child. The milk we drink on the other hand, which has been processed and then delivered to us after some time gap is acidic. Not that our digestive machinery cannot digest this milk. It very well can, our machinery is so strong that it can break down some of the toughest substances, but at what cost? At the cost of consumption of massive amounts of brain energy! The energy which, if free and available for other purposes can make you feel like a Super Hero. So yes, the milk with acidic properties can also be digested but with massive consumption of energy. Saliva is the catalyst which can convert this acid into alkaline, making it soft on our digestive machinery and conserving a lot of energy in the process. Fletcherising makes this happen. It does the same to all kinds of juices, tea, coffee and other drinks. It makes them sober, softer, digestion friendly.

How do we Fletcherise milk and other liquids? It's the way wine tasters taste wine says Fletcher. They don't drink wine, they smell it, they sip it, and they taste it making sure they get the most out of every sip.

Of course milk wouldn't probably smell as good as wine but if you love milk, the taste will be worth the effort. It's the same with any other drink, soups or any other food in a liquid form. Taking smaller sips and allowing them to disappear into the throat or kind of absorbed into the mouth, instead of "Drinking" it "bottoms up", reveals a kind of delicious mouth watering taste even in the simplest of the drinks, a taste not hitherto experienced. I never noticed in the past, watering of the mouth while drinking milk or tea or coffee. But now when I sip I realize the taste buds are as excited to receive these sumptuous liquids as they are to receive the delicious foods. The taste buds welcome every sip with an ample supply of saliva.

Water, if it is at the room temperature, does not need to be parked in the mouth as food and other drinks have to be. It does seem to halt a little though when one is not very thirsty. If the water is too hot or too cold, we do feel the initial resistance as soon as the water touches any part of our mouth. The Food Filter shuts down. It is a sign like all the other signs we keep receiving. It will do only good to respect this sign and hold the water in the mouth for a while, and then pass it on once it feels normal. Water does taste good though if we notice a bit. No other drink is as tasty as water is. Nothing quenches the thirst for water, but water!

When, How, What and How much to drink is again something every individual needs to decide based on his appetite, her thirst in the moment.

When, What, How and How Much

Soup and other food in liquid form is not a drink, but is food. These can be had in response to the appetite as has been discussed previously. Tea, coffee, juices or any other drink again is driven by appetite and not by thirst alone. Water is the only drink called for by thirst. So water can be had in response to thirst, evidenced by drying of the mouth and other drinks can be taken in response to ones appetite.

There are several theories doing rounds about how much of water one needs to drink–8 glasses, 10 glasses, 1 liter, 2 liters. Fletcherism does not prescribe any quantity. What is true for food is true for water. Drink as much as is required to quench the thirst and not to fill up the stomach. As for the other drinks–tea, coffee, milk, wine, alcoholic drinks, drink as much as is permitted by the appetite but Fletcherise–like the Wine Tasters Taste Wine! Having said that, it will be noticed eventually that Nature's favorite drink is water only! Nature prescribes water over, and instead of, all other drinks. But this statement again is something that you don't have to force yourself to believe in. You can let the "Water find its own level" like it is with every aspect of Fletcherising.

Like overeating, drinking more water than is required by the body, also leads to experiencing heaviness in the stomach and wastage in the form of frequent urination and sweating. Come to think of it, agreed it takes much less energy for the body to process the excess of water to get rid of it, and the damage done is also not as severe as in case of overeating, it still is a waste of energy to some degree. A waste we can easily avoid with the expert guidance of Nature.

On whether we should or should not drink water between meals, immediately before or after meals, and does it interfere with digestion, Fletcher notes: "*Water injures digestion by being taken with meals only because it is used to wash down food not yet prepared for the stomach. It is the unfit food that is carried down by it and not the water that does the harm.*" I used to drink at least a glassful of water between meals, one because I did feel thirsty and two, thinking it is somehow aiding digestion and helping move the food through the digestive track and further through bowels. However since I started Fletcherising, from day one, I don't take even a sip of water between meals and just a couple of sips after meals. This again like every other change was natural and not a forced or conscious choice. The understanding that all the natural bodily processes are, by their very Nature free flowing, and that one does not have to help "push" the flow, dawns upon every Fletcherite, sooner than later. Furthermore the secretion and intake of saliva in ample quantity makes sure his body and mouth remains more hydrated and he does not feel thirsty that often. And this is not just only between meals but also at all other times.

3

Saliva–The Elixir of life

Elixir, in the Dictionary, is defined as "a magical potion, especially one supposedly able to make people live forever". Saliva has been scientifically proven to have several healing and digestive properties. Its chemical properties are such that for a person from a nonscientific background, it takes some efforts to even pronounce them right. In a layman's term, Saliva is the Elixir of Life, the Elixir pursued by the Alchemists without, but which was always within! It may not make you live forever (or may be it may, we can't be sure), but it certainly helps you live longer by neutralizing the harmful, fatty, acidic, bacteria infected substances that enter the body through the mouth. That is if we allow these substances to remain in contact with the Saliva for a longer period of time. That is if we Fletcherise!

On this subject Fletcher says: *Nature has a good reason for everything she plans. It is asserted by physiological chemists that saliva, taken from the mouth and kept at normal temperature, will dissolve breads and similar foods and convert the starch in them into maltose, glucose or sugar. The converted form is that which is suitable for further digestion. Saliva also converts some acids into alkali and readily neutralizes all acids.*

Saliva is not just for lubrication or moistening of the food in order to render it easy to swallow. It is the greatest "digestive" ever produced.

There was this article I read in the local newspaper (which by the way is the article which got me started on Fletcherism), which spoke about how Saliva aids in Digestion, "*Digestion begins in our mouth. Efficient chewing increases the surface area of foods, affording a thorough breakdown by enzymes. Saliva also contains lingual lipase, a fat metabolizing enzyme, which breaks down fat before it reaches the stomach. If the fat reached the stomach inadequately chewed, brace yourself for digestion problems. The longer our food stays in touch with our saliva, the better it gets lubricated and lesser the stress on our esophagus. Even digesting carbohydrates starts with chewing right as our saliva detaches chemical bonds that connect the starch containing simple sugars. When you don't chew well, these enzymes can't break down starches or digest fats, inducing sluggishness and loss of energy*"

Saliva has scientifically proven healing properties. It's not too much to say that the constant supply of saliva into our body is what keeps us fit and healed to a very large extent. There is this Bible story where Jesus mixed saliva with mud and applied it to a man's eyes. There is scientific evidence now to support the actions of Jesus. Saliva is a very effective healing agent and can help treat skin and eye conditions. Saliva contains a chemical that aids in the speedy healing of wounds. A quick browsing of internet on properties of saliva will give truck loads of evidences and reports proving why Saliva is really the Elixir of Life.

There are many who suffer from the Dry Mouth Syndrome where the natural secretion of saliva is either very low or completely absent. This happens, in some cases as a side effect of various medical treatments like Chemotherapy which destroy or render partially dysfunctional the salivary glands, and in many cases due to a plain underutilization or non-utilization of this very important Nature given apparatus. No one understands the value of Saliva as much as those who have a limited supply or no supply at all of this natural liquid. In any case, Fletcherising is worth a try. It encourages secretion of saliva. Keeping the food for a longer while in the mouth will help the taste buds do their job and motivate the salivary glands to do their bit. Why, Fletcherising could also act as a preventive measure to the Dry Mouth Syndrome! Like a body which is constantly kept active remains healthier than the one which is inactive, the Salivary Glands of a Fletcherite will be in a much healthier condition than those of a non Fletcherite.

Fletcherising enables production and utilization of this Elixir in abundance ensuring a healthier life to begin with!

4

Fletcherism–Summary

"The proof of the pudding is in the eating" goes the saying. This may not be entirely true for a Fletcherite. A Fletcherite eats, not for the love of food but out of the love for self! Having said that, no one else can do as much justice to the pudding, as the Fletcherite can!

The type of food set in front of a Fletcherite will not drive his appetite or impact the pleasure she gets out of the food. A Fletcherite enjoys every type of food that is called for by his appetite.

As is noted about Fletcher in the book "The New Glutton or Epicure", *"Fletcher eat **just what his appetite called for**, as nearly as circumstances of supply permitted, he ate all **that his appetite would allow**; enjoyed a gustatory pleasure that **had never been equaled** under the old habits of taking food, and was a distinct epicurean gainer by the economy learned and practiced. But—and in this "but" lies the secret—the solid food had been munched appreciatively until it was liquefied and a strong Swallowing Impulse compelled its deglutition. The sapid and nutritious liquids were tasted as the wine tasters taste wine, as the tea tasters taste tea, and as all experts test, or "Get the Good" out of anything. Instead of being drunk down in a flood like water, which has no taste and no reason to stay in the region of taste, delicious country milk was sipped and tasted with the end of the tongue, where the best taste buds are, until it disappeared by natural absorption.*

This is what Fletcherising is all about, technically–chewing your drinks and drinking your foods!

This process is made easy with the help of all the natural tools that was given to us, by Nature, to be utilized. What happens inside the body is something which we cannot see. It would be very cruel on the part of the Creator to expect us to see and understand what is happening in there, but Nature is not cruel. Nature has done all it could to make it easy for us in the form of these visible signs like hunger, appetite, the basic design of the mouth–the teeth, saliva, flexible structure of the jaws, the parking lots, the natural food filter and the taste buds.

How good or bad the couple of chocolate bars you have every day is? How harmful or harmless the packets of crisps you have in a week are? How healthy or unhealthy the cheese cakes and cheese pizzas are? How necessary or unnecessary the multiple meals we have in a day are? How appropriate or inappropriate the quantity of food we consume is? How adequate or inadequate the nutrition we have through our food is? What is the right quantity of water we should be drinking in a day? Do we need to drink anything other than water? Do we need to eat raw vegetables? Do we need to eat meat? No one outside of us can answer these questions for us. Our body, the inbuilt, God given mechanism in it knows these answers and does keep guiding us.

One doesn't need to analyze scientifically the cravings of the body. One doesn't need to have the understanding of the subject of Anatomy to interpret the purpose each organ in the body was meant to serve to assist the voluntary act of eating and drinking. One does not need to know the scientific properties of Saliva to make it work. It still works! The entire apparatus works even if we don't know how it does. We just need to fulfill our role in the process. There is only one pre-requisite to get started, the willingness to Fletcherise sincerely.

As Fletcher puts it, "*Any person can employ Dr. Normal Appetite and consult Dr. Good Taste **free of all charge,** and make endless discoveries in the possibility of delightful and healthfully economic nutrition*"

5

Perfect Weight

When I started Fletcherising, I was about 25 to 30 pounds overweight. The sudden weight loss (all of the excess weight) in 15 weeks was a surprise to everyone and even to me since I had not expected the results this fast. As with any exercise routine or diet, I was probably expecting only about an inch of reduction here and there, a couple of pounds of weight loss in the initial couple of months. And maybe over a period of a year, I would have imagined losing about 10 to 15 pounds and then probably back to square one after a while when I get back to my old eating habits. Little did I know I was changing my eating habits for a life time in these 15 weeks. Furthermore how can that which was true for Horace Fletcher, the Legendary Health Guru, be true for me, a layman, who didn't know and was not very interested in "right eating", me, who has never been a fitness freak, me, who has always eaten for pleasure only, not giving the slightest of the thoughts to the "nutritional" aspect of any food or drink, me, *who lived to eat!*

Fletcherism worked and continues to work for me, the way it worked for Fletcher and so it can work for anybody and everybody!

It's for Both–the Over weights and the Under Weights

I was overweight so Fletcherising helped me reduce weight but for those who are underweight, it will help gain some weight. Fletcher

27

conducted an experiment on some ordinary Tramps picked up in the streets of Chicago. He notes that there were fat and thin among them. They were taught how to Fletcherise and they did. It was surprising to see that after some time into it, some of those who were thin put on weight and those who were fat lost weight at the same time.

The ones who are lean or maybe even underweight need not worry that Fletcherising will make them even skinnier. It will not, they can try it for themselves and see how it helps them gain weight.

It may not bring you to the "Natural weight" as prescribed in medical journals or health publications. By that standard, a Fletcherite may be a couple of pounds overweight or underweight. But does that matter? I am about 5 pounds underweight when I look at the standards set for my height. I am 162 cm in height so should be about 110 to 115 pounds in weight. I am about 106 pounds now, so technically speaking, I am underweight but Naturally speaking, I am at my perfect weight, the weight prescribed by Nature!

Food is Good

I always thought it was food that made me overweight, the type of food I eat—oily, buttery, spicy, all the so called comfort foods, all the different type of chocolates, biscuits and cakes on the shelves of the grocery stores that caught my attention, all the cheese and milk I consumed as a routine. It took about more than a couple of months of Fletcherising for me to realize it is not the food. It never was the food. It's not the food that makes us overweight. It's not the food which gives that bloated feeling. It's not the food that causes constipation. It's not the food that makes us feel tired, lazy, inactive, diseased, and completely hopeless in a nutshell, at times. Food, in whatever form it is in, is not the bad guy here, it cannot be, Food is Good!

Food has been considered a form of divinity in several religions. Food has been treated with respect and reverence in ancient traditions, why even today, in many homes, a prayer of thanks giving is offered at the table, for the food. I was born into a Hindu family where food is considered a form of God. I got married into a Roman Catholic family and understood it was the same there as well. There is this statement written in bible, that Jesus Christ made. Jesus, at his last supper, said that the bread was his body and the wine his blood. Keeping religion aside I interpreted this statement as; food is the body of Christ, the body of the son of God, body of God. God is pure love, God is divine. The body of God is also pure love in that case, it is divine. So food is pure love, food is divine. That which is pure love only nourishes and gives life. It doesn't know what else to do. Why else would Christ say the food is his body and wine is his blood, why else would almost all religions consider food as sacred and meal time as auspicious.

Meal time is one of the best times in the day and most of us really look forward to it. Food comforts and nourishes, it gives a kind of happiness very few things can give, it keeps us alive! It is one of the most wonderful gifts given to us by the Creator.

If we underutilize or mis-utilize this love, this nourishment, we are depriving ourselves of all the good it can do to us. Unconditional love as I theoretically understand is giving away the best that you have to the other without expecting anything in return. It's like the sun giving away its best—the sunshine, warmth, radiance, light. It's like the flowers giving away the best they have—fragrance and beauty. Likewise food, in any form only gives the best it has, nourishment and nutrition. Every bite of food comes with this gift of love and nourishment. The giver of the gift is giving its unconditional gift, now if the receiver is not receiving it with love, one can't blame the giver. A pack of crisp is not bad—it contains fat, calories, carbohydrates, sugar, starch, some proteins, vitamins and minerals maybe nowadays. All of this, everyone will agree, is required by the body. It's just that the body may not need it at a particular time or maybe the body does need all these at that time, but not in the quantity in which we put it into our body. In what proportion and at what times is what needs understanding. A Fletcherite would know this. Fletcherising makes sure this gift of food is made use of in all the beautiful ways in which it was intended to be made use of.

Likewise drinks, be it water, juices, milk or any other drink are all sources of nourishment. Anything that we put into our body has to go there with love, reverence and acceptance and this can be done only by thoroughly Fletcherising everything that passes through our mouth.

No food is bad. No food by itself can cause any harm to our health and well being. Blaming the food for our ill heath is like blaming alcohol for the state of an alcoholic. Alcohol in itself is not bad, it has medicinal properties, and it is used in medicines. It's not the alcohol that is the curse, it's the conscious decision of the alcoholic—it's an incorrect choice—incorrect with regard to the "when and how much to put into the body"!

The tug of war between vegetarians and non vegetarians never seems to end. It also has been given a religious tone at times. Some religions don't mind the followers eating meat and drinking wine whereas there are others where consumption of meat or wine is forbidden. The way I see it there is nothing religious about food and drinks. Food is just good food and a drink is just a good drink. If I don't wish to have a particular type of food or drink, that's my personal choice, God does not judge me based on what I eat. God does not judge me anyways. The type of food and drinks consumed differ from one country to another, from one locality to another, from one family, one individual to another. Fletcherism does not set any standard; there is no right or wrong food here. What does go wrong is the demand supply timing and quantity—the demands of the body and the conscious supply of food by our own choice. If the best of the foods rich in all the vitamins, minerals and proteins is put into the body at a time when the body does not need it and in an un-Fletcherised form, then the food and eventually our health is as good as wasted.

6

Radiant Health

It was not with the sole aim of losing weight that I had started Fletcherising. Rather weight loss was only somewhere at the back of my mind. What fascinated me was what Fletcherism could do to my physical strength and endurance, my stamina and immunity. The energy and vigor it promised seemed to be a dream come true. And all this without sweating my life out at a Gym or reluctantly doing a sport or adopting an exercise routine.

I have started taking about 25 minute walks though, everyday, but this is only because my body feels so active that it does not want to be sitting and lazing around after I come home from a day's desk work. Since past couple of months rather my body tells me to go out and get some fresh air even in the mornings which I have never done ever before but enjoy doing now.

Fletcherism indeed has been and continues to be the best gift I could give to my physical self. This hitherto neglected area of my life is now totally sorted!

Fletcherism is not just about Weight Management

Fletcherism is not just a weight management tool. Weight management is an essential by product and the very first physical sign of the fact that it is working its magic on you. Before I started Fletcherising, I was at a stage where I was sick of feeling tired every evening, of the heaviness in my legs, my body. I was beginning to get worried about the state of my health because of the lack of exercise and dietary control.

Fletcherising was the only method, I ever came across, which was all about eating but did not tell me that I need to include salads or fruits or this liquid or that solid in my diet or that I should give up any of my favorite foods. This did not tell me that I needed to exercise for 30 minutes every day at least 4 days a week etc. I immediately took to the idea because I have always loved food and hated "forced exercising" even if it was I forcing myself. I was thoroughly impressed with the findings of the experiments conducted on and by Horace Fletcher. The level of strength and endurance Fletcher demonstrated was kind of unbelievable and would be a dream come true if it worked for me.

There are these couple of tests, out of the many that Fletcher went through to test his strength and endurance. Reading these and the others put me in awe and I knew I had to Fletcherise.

Fletcher writes: "*Two years after I began my experiments my strength and endurance had increased beyond my wildest expectation. On my fiftieth birthday I rode nearly two hundred miles on my bicycle over French roads, and came home feeling fine. Was I stiff the next day? Not at all, and I rode fifty miles the next morning before breakfast in order to test the effect of my severe stunt.*

When I was fifty eight years of age, at the Yale University Gymnasium, under the observation of Dr. Anderson. I Lifted three hundred pounds dead weight three hundred and fifty times with the muscles of my right leg below the knee."

And it's worth noting that the record of the best athlete, then at the Yale University Gymnasium was one hundred and seventy five lifts. Fletcher had doubled the world's record of that style of tests of endurance.

Now this is impressive, very impressive! Anyone who is not Fletcherising but can pull this kind of a stunt off is a genuine Super

Man. Anyone who cannot, needs to Fletcherise! I cannot yet do this, so Fletcherising is what I will continue to do.

This increase in strength and endurance of a Fletcherite is not something Science cannot explain. There is very little or even no waste, eventually, generated in the body since the nutritional intake is just right. There are no toxins running around in the blood stream, in the muscles, tissues and bones. Every cell of the body is as pure as Nature designed it to be. The Brain energy hitherto consumed in the process of digestion, assimilation and distribution is freed up and utilized to assist rest of the bodily functions. And when you are Fletcherising, following the Natures way, you receive Natures abundant and unlimited rewards, both in mind and body.

So if there is someone out there who is "technically" lean and fit with "healthy eating habits" and so thinks, "Fletcherising is not for me", it would help to assess his or her own level of strength and endurance and compare it with that reflected in the experiments above. I did question initially, "Okay it worked for Horace Fletcher, but will it work for me?" I got the answer in the first 5 months. My story has a stark resemblance with Fletchers. If what 5 months of Fletcherising did to me was the same as what it did to Fletcher, the same peak of strength, health and endurance is mine to have as well. These goodies are up for grabs for everyone!

As I have mentioned earlier, the resultant weight loss was a surprise because I was not looking at that, the aim was and is, perfect radiant health! Everything else falls into place in perfect harmony.

So Fletcherism is a Universal cure for everyone, the lean, the fat, the tall, the short, the fit, the unfit, the healthy the unhealthy, the strong and the weak, the rich and the poor, the child, the adult, the aged, every single one!

Beautiful Within, Beautiful Without

Fletcher has conducted several experiments and noted the findings on the impact of Fletcherising on the waste generated and thrown out from the body. It is fascinating to read that any waste generated out of a Fletcherites body will have no offensive odor, be it the digestion ash (excreta), urine or sweat. Nothing about him will ever stink! She may use a perfume only because she likes the fragrance and not because she may smell bad in case she sweats. A Fletcherites toilet can never be unclean or polluted.

The impurities within is what creates the impurities without. The Fletcherites body will be so clean within that there will be no need to take a lot of efforts to keep it clean without. The beauty or antiseptic soaps, all the cleansing lotions and potions may still be used but only out of sheer habit or because these products smell good or feel good, but there will be no need to really cleanse the body using any of these tools. There will be no impurity which needs forced cleaning. Natural cleansing–Fletcherising will take care of this.

Unbalanced nutritional intake is also known to cause several problems such as hair fall, dandruff, dull hair, pimples, acne, blemishes on the skin, dark circles and many such "beauty issues". These are all the symptoms of undernourished or incorrectly fed body. Fletcherising puts this in balance which will automatically take care of all these issues. Fletcherising restores the natural, healthy, blemish free glow that is seen on the skin of a baby, it puts the hair and scalp back to its natural state of health. It would not be too much to imagine that our skin will eventually become so aligned with Nature that whatever be the season, it will acclimatize itself to the changing seasons without there being any need to take care externally by applying the lotions and potions. For example the skin may not dry up during winters or become oily during summers, the hair also may retain its natural shine irrespective of the climatic conditions.

It's too early for me to have experienced this complete internal cleansing since I understand that all the garbage collected in about 30 years time may not be completely wiped off and destroyed in a few months of Fletcherising. But I know I am getting there because:

1) I don't feel as bloated as I used to. Rather I feel a bit bloated only on the days I have been a little bad and indulged not

heeding Natures signs. It could be more of a mental than a physical feeling I believe since I am so used to feeling light now a days that even the slightest deviation makes me stand up and notice. These days would have gone thoroughly unnoticed in the past.

2) My skin, in the past, would get oily end of the day because probably I had an oily skin I thought. But now it doesn't, it remains as fresh as it was in the morning.

3) My skin feels softer than ever before. It still has spots and dots which I am sure will disappear eventually

4) My beautician says that my blackheads have reduced noticeably

5) I used to apply lotions and potions all year round to keep my skin soft and moistened. I haven't done that in the last five months, I may have to do it now in winter but eventually I think I can get rid of this need completely

6) The quantity of perfumes and deodorants I used to apply has also reduced; I somehow know now its okay to keep it to bare minimum.

Well this is just the beginning and I know there are much more surprises in stock for the one walking on the path of Fletcherism. Fletcherism in this sense is the Nature Assigned Beautician who constantly keeps you beautiful within and so beautiful without!

My Friend with Hypo-thyroid and Those with Other Ailments

One of my friends suffers from Hypo-thyroid. The major symptoms she was suffering from were fatigue, depression, weight gain. She has been on medication for several years, both Homeopathy and Allopathic to keep her weight regulated, to help her stay above depression and fatigue. These medicines did keep her weight from increasing rapidly and also kept a check on depression. She however felt too lazy to be active. A few minutes' walk would tire her and she would want to stop it and go home. It was around the mid of May, 2012 when I met her and we chatted about Fletcherism. She took to it right away. Three months into it and she called to tell me that she had lost about 17 pounds. She now enjoyed walking more than ever, she would walk for 5 minutes, and would feel like walking some more and then some more. Her doctor also noticed the change and asked what she has been up to. She said it was Fletcherising and her Doctor encouraged her to continue. She has been advised to skip the medicines once a week–every Sunday. This was the physical change, what happened to her fatigue and depression? Well fatigue is gone as well, and depression, why would anyone who was overweight, tired and not very healthy be depressed anymore with such an easy to use and effective cure at hand?

Even if we do not analyze it with scientific accuracy, it is apparent that Fletcherising is neutralizing one of the major symptoms of Hypo-thyroid–weight gain. So it would not be completely wrong to assume that if it can neutralize the symptoms, it can neutralize the ailment itself.

It's too soon to assess probably if she can do away completely with her medicines which helped her stay at a constant weight, I wouldn't be surprised to find out from her after another two months or maybe couple of more months that she has stopped taking medicines altogether and that her ailment has completely disappeared.

For me this is a miracle, a well founded, scientifically provable, Natures miracle. A miracle which will work for everyone without exception, Fletcherism cannot fail!

This for me, gives hope to all those who suffer from any ailment, be it those with diabetes, any of the heart diseases or those with cancer or fibroids or tumors in any of their organs. The imbalance of sugar, starch, cholesterol or any other substance or fluid in the body is largely on account of incorrect eating and so can be cured by correct eating. All these ailments, the cancerous cells or fibroids and tumors in the body derive their strength from either the lack of or the excess of any of the body fluids or chemicals, from the toxins in the body, the waste generated, something which is in excess than that which is required by the body, or something which is less than that the body requires. Food and drinks are the most important causes of this excess or dearth. Once this supply is set right and the body is balanced in all ways, these unwanted cancerous cells cannot prosper, multiply, become strong or even stay alive for that matter.

On this Fletcher says, *"It is said that none of the microbes of disease can live an instant, and hence cannot propagate, in a perfectly healthy human tissue. It is possible to secure the perfectly healthy human tissue, to both the generally healthy and to those who are afflicted, unless too far gone to reform, by keen attention to the direction of Taste, and the reward of the attention is manifold. The actual pleasure derived from eating under the direction of the method suggested herein cannot be equaled by any other means."*

This amazing master piece of the creator, our body, is so wonderfully strong and persistent in its life wards journey that it strives to an extent which is beyond our imagination to keep us alive and going. It never gives up on us. It just constantly keeps on keeping on. That's the reason the symptoms of ill health start showing up for most only after the initial 20 to 25 years of our lives. It starts with subtler signs such as indigestion, headaches, frequent coughs and colds, muscle pulls, cramps, fatigue, laziness and so on.

Nowadays however this shows up earlier, even in children. Children with diabetes were an unheard of occurrence in the past which now is increasing in proportion. One can argue how can that be since children don't generally misuse the liberty given by Nature that early. No the children don't, but their parents have, it's the parents body, that passes on to the child with all its purities or impurities. The child comes with these impurities inherited. How else can we explain the "family history" of heart disease and diabetes and cancer? There is hope though even if you are one of these inherent carriers of disease, you can stop it in your generation so that the generations ahead or for that matter you in your own life time don't have to live with this "family history".

Fletcherising keeps a check on the waste generated in the body keeping it pure. Where the waste generated in the body eventually lowers, the strength of these cancerous cells, fibroids and diseased cells also diminishes as they don't have enough poison to feed on and they cannot live on pure nourishment. Our healthy cells cannot live on poison; likewise these poisonous cells cannot live on healthy food. Fletcherising furthermore adds to the strength of healthy cells by supplying the right nutrition. So the inbuilt healing mechanism of the body gets all the more powerful and reaches a state where all the diseased cells are either destroyed or made healthy again.

I am not suggesting that anyone with one of these serious ailments should skip their medicines or experiment with their diets. Fletcherism can be practiced even with the existing prescribed diets. Only one change is called for to begin with, masticating thoroughly whatever it is that you are eating. Eventually, like my friend, there may be lesser and lesser need to rely on any healing tool outside of you.

Strength and Endurance

Most of us are living in a body which is biologically several years older than our age. Do we really know how a really healthy body feels, the energy, the strength, the endurance, the lightness, the bounciness, the springiness? How would it feel to be bouncing around and running around like little children do without the fear of any resultant dislocation of one of the bones or a muscle pull or a cramp or soreness the next day? How would it feel to climb up a flight of stairs, no matter how tall the building, and arrive at the terrace with breath as normal and body as fresh and energetic as when you started? How would it feel to go hiking and never get tired, not at the start and not at the end? How would it feel to be really what is called "Hale and Hearty"?

Fletcherism produces visible results from the very first day in the quantity of food consumed and the way the stomach feels after the meal. However the level of strength and endurance demonstrated by Fletcher and others in the experiments recorded in the books noted earlier is not something that was achieved in a day, week or even a month. These experiments do prove though what a Fletcherite can expect as long term benefit (sooner than later) of this new formed habit of Fletcherising.

"Fletcherism–what is it and how I became young at 60" talks about the tests of endurance conducted by Professor Irving Fisher, of Yale with the cooperation of the famous athletic coach, Alonzo B. Stagg, on College athletes, students of sedentary habits, and on members of the staff of the Battle Creek Sanatorium. These, some other experiments and the notes of Fletcher noted below prove what Fletcherism can do to ones physical strength and endurance:

a) *These tests are of prodigious importance in their relation to the possibilities of human endurance through simple Fletcherising. The reports include a test in what is termed "deep knee bending," or squatting on the heels and then lifting the body to full height as many times as possible. John H. Granger, of the Battle Creek Sanatorium staff, did this feat 5,002 times consecutively in two hours and nineteen minutes and could have continued. He then ran down a flight of steps to the swimming pool, plunged in and had a swim, slept sweetly and soundly for the usual time, and showed no signs of soreness or other disability afterwards.*

b) *Doctor Wagner gave his strenuous contribution to our knowledge of possibilities of endurance by holding his arms out horizontally for 200 minutes without rest—three hours and twenty minutes. At the end of that time he showed no signs of fatigue, and stopped only because of the weariness shown by those who were watching and counting the minutes. These statements seem like exaggerations, but they are not. Both of these tests can be tried by anyone in the privacy of his or her own bedroom.*

c) *Doctor Anderson, Director of the Yale Gymnasium, taking advantage of the cue offered by the Yale experiments, which he superintended, practiced Fletcherising in all its branches. At the end of six years he put the muscles thus purified to the test, with the result that he added fifteen pounds of pure muscle to a frame that never carried more than 135 pounds before in the half century of its existence, and demonstrated that the same progressive recuperation that I have enjoyed is open and available to others who have passed middle life.*

d) When Fletcher did about 304 kilometers of cycling on his 50th birthday, he notes that "*it was a revelation of possibilities to a man of fifty who had once, not many years before, been denied life insurance on account of health disability. This was worth more*

> *than millions of money to me; and no one knows how much it will signify to the human family when the knowledge of a truly economic nutrition is attained and established."*

e) In another experiment conducted by Fletcher on his muscle strength and endurance after a long period of inaction, he notes, *"Once, after nearly a year of physical inactivity, I took with me an attendant and made an average of seventy five miles a day in the mountain districts of southern Germany for observation of increase of food requirement during hard work. Neither muscular soreness, nor muscular fatigue, except the periodical weariness of sleepiness, were experienced as the result of the sudden change from the most restful environment to strenuous activity; and herein lies a physiological question that is far reaching in its significance. It would seem that Appetite, in its normal condition, assisted in its discrimination by careful mouth treatment of food, guards the body from excess and keeps it always "in training".*

These and several other experiments conducted by Fletcher on self, on others and those conducted by others on Fletcher and other Fletcherites prove the authenticity of the results Fletcherism promises to deliver. I must add a word of caution here though. Couple of months into Fletcherising will not give the body the level of strength and endurance revealed here in the experiments and so one should not try performing feats of very adventurous nature. There will of course be this temptation to put to test the newfound energy and vigor, which one can do, but in small ways. The limit to which you wish to stretch yourself is purely left to your discretion.

My strength and endurance levels are nowhere close to that demonstrated in the experiments above but I know for sure I am headed in that direction because of the increase in energy and stamina that I experience.

Every Fletcherite can get to the peak of physical strength and endurance demonstrated in the experiments above, sooner than later, just that every person is different from the other and the time involved in the process will differ.

As is noted in Fletchers books, "*Fletcher has voluminous data relative to his work, but it is not applicable to any other person. Each person is a law unto himself and no two sets of conditions are alike. **Treat your food as advised herein and get surprising new experiences for yourselves, is the advice and moral of the story.***"

Looking Younger, Youthful old age and Long life

As noted previously, we are all living in a body which is biologically a bit older than our chronological age. With Fletcherising, my personal experience has been that I have started looking younger (I always felt younger but now I also look younger). I felt very good when I was told by my friends that I don't look like the middle aged grown up woman I used to look like and that I looked like a college going girl now. It feels good to be receiving such complements and when these come from more than one source, you have to trust the authenticity of the compliments. It's not just looking younger and good that matters, of course this matters, but what matters more than this is the fact that when you Fletcherise, you restore your body to the right biological age. It's not that Fletcherising is an anti–aging agent which reduces your age, it doesn't. It only makes sure that the body's wear and tear is minimized and that it is restored to the state of health it was supposed to be in the first place. Yes, this is the way my body was supposed to look in the first place as per the "Default Factory Settings" but somewhere because of the customizations (I mean eating and not the beauty products etc.), things went wrong. I am 32 years old, I never felt this mentally as I was always my mammas little girl, but I did look like a 32 year old grown up. I don't look 32 anymore, I now look like my mammas "college going" little girl!

Fletcher narrates the story of a patriarch who at sixty five, was awaiting death with constant expectancy and was trying to attain it by every sort of favorable suggestion, "*He had his portrait taken in a photograph gallery on his sixty fifth birthday as a last souvenir to be distributed among his friends. Shortly after that, he met with "accidental" suggestion (Fletcherism) which changed his habits of living, and, very soon, his attitude toward life and death. I sat with the patriarch on his one hundredth birthday in the same photograph gallery, examined the portraits of sixty five and one hundred years,* conversed with the subject in a low tone of voice, looked upon a man who felt that he was yet in middle life, and in possession of an enjoyment of life that he said had never been equaled in the early years of his bondage to the ignorance and impatience of youth"

The Patriarch lived for 100+ years, and would you not like to? There are some who say they don't want to be that old and want to live just for about 50 or 60 years, they fear old age as it were, but if the old age comes without any signs of old age, would you mind hanging around for 100, 150 or even more years in the pink of your health? All those in old age and in good, radiant state of health are decent eaters, Fletcherites to a very great extent.

Fletcherism alone does not guarantee long life though; it increases the probability by keeping you in the best of health. Fletcher died at the age of 69 because of Bronchitis. How could Fletcher have Bronchitis? And how could he die at the age of 69? I don't want to know. What I do want to know is how he lived his life, the state of radiant health he was in, the work he did which has touched lives, changed lives! He started Fletcherising at the age of 40, so enjoyed robust health and lived life fully for about 29 years. He has attained a legendary status and has been immortalized in these 29 years. As the saying goes, "It's not the years in life but the life in the years that matters". If my previous lifestyle would have given me say x number of years to live, I am sure Fletcherising will give me x+ years which, in terms of the life in it will be worth more than at least double of what the previous lifestyle would have given. And maybe that's what would have happened to Fletcher as well. Had he not started Fletcherising at 40, he might have passed away way before the age of 69 going by the state of health he was in at the age of 40.

So yes Fletcherising does increase the years in your life and also the life in your years!

Specially for Women

"Health is Wealth", this is true equally for Men and Women. For Women there is this additional need to be extra fit because of the way

God has created us and because of the role our body plays in bringing a new life into the world. Menstruation cycles and Pregnancy are the two areas of a woman's life where Fletcherising can provide comfort and make it easy and even blissful for the women to go through.

Menstruation:

Fletcherising can help get rid of all the pain and discomfort women suffer during their periods. It's not just a long term benefit; the change is noticeable right away from the very first month from what I experienced. The laziness, the tired feeling, the cramps, the pain in the abdomen and lower back, the bloated feeling, irritable bowel movements, the gases, the weakness and even for the matter the irritable moods women go through during these days is minimized and even completely eliminated eventually.

There is this need the body has during these days, to rest, to slow down. Many women lose their appetite and the food intake is also reduced. Maybe it's a sign again from the Nature (one out of the many that Nature keeps sending and we keep ignoring) to stop and notice what is going on. A nudge to make appropriate changes in our lifestyle, our eating habits, to take stock of whether they are helping us stay healthy or are damaging our natural bodily processes. Fletcherism is a preventive measure to avoid all these unpleasant experiences associated with menstruation.

With Fletcherising, partially because of the sudden weight loss and the change in food intake, in the initial couple of months, there could be some irregularities in terms of the flow and the dates. It is as if the body is rebooting its systems after a very long time and often for the first time since we developed teeth and learnt to eat wrong. The processes and programs in here which run this magnificent, fully automated, wonderful machine of ours get reset. They are restored to the "Default Factory Settings". It is but obvious then that there will be some noise, some downtime, some rescheduling. This is a very positive sign and nothing to be worried about.

If changes are occurring and it starts to worry you, try and look at how you actually feel about it, not think about it, but feel about it. Thinking, analyzing and calculating is good where it comes to numbers but when we talk about ourselves, our bodies, our minds and our lives, what we feel about all this is the only important bit. For me personally, I did go through this rebooting, resetting and restarting phase. Thinking did make it look bad, but I felt all was going good. I felt nice and healthy. There was no outward sign like uneasiness or pain or any discomfort of any sort that may indicate something could be going wrong. So I kept the faith and carried on. It was all okay eventually in a couple of month's time.

Blissful pregnancy

The most common first signs of a woman being pregnant are missing periods and throwing up. Missing periods is understandable but why throwing up? The throwing up continues for most women during the first 3 months and for some throughout the 9 months. Is not throwing up connected completely in one way or the other to the food or water or any other drink in the stomach? At least that's what comes out when you throw up–food, water, any other drink mixed with the various digestive juices and liquids in our stomach. Doctors say this is because of the hormonal changes that take place when you are pregnant. Whatever be the scientific, logical and analytical explanation to the phenomenon of a pregnant women throwing up, it's worth giving a thought about what is on the Creators mind? What is Nature up to here? It seems so much like sign again to an expectant mother from the Creator, a reminder from Nature that there is a new life coming into this world through you, so take care of what you put in there, into your body, into your stomach, for the one who has just physically arrived into your womb.

The Natural instincts are at its peak in an expectant mother. There is nothing strange then, that pregnant women suddenly crave for some food they may never have fancied eating before or they even give up on things they so loved, not forcefully, but naturally, they just don't want to eat any more the food that they so loved a couple of months ago. There is this new life taking form within, a life that is so close, so one with Nature, whose basic blue print is intact, untouched, untainted by habits, methods and customizations of the world outside. This new life reaches out to the mum to be, urging her to align to Natures plan and design and hence the sudden change in the eating habits.

Why should pregnancy, Gods best gift to women, be anything less than blissful? Why should there be any unpleasant experience or feeling of discomfort associated with this phase of life? The unpleasant experiences such as throwing up, dizziness, weakness, strength and endurance issues, the swelling of body, excess weight gain (over and above the normal weight gain expected during these days), problems with digestion, increase / decrease in blood pressure, sugar levels, thyroid levels—are they an essential part of pregnancy? Of course there are hormonal changes, the requirements of the body changes but can they not be nice and easy, like every natural process, can't pregnancy be an enjoyable and blissful experience with not even a trace of discomfort on any single day, be it the First, Second or Third Trimester? Child birth again, why does it have to be painful? Why does Child Birth have to be "Push!!!! Breathe!!!!Push!!!!Breathe !!!!…." with a lot of pain involved in the process? Why can't it be, relax, breathe easy, and the baby just slides out, giving its mommy the most blissful experience of her life.

If I or anyone has to name the one thing that is most important during pregnancy and can take care of most of the pregnancy related issues, it would be "right nutrition". The second important thing is strength and endurance which is majorly an outcome of "right nutrition". The third important thing which matters the most during child birth is the level of flexibility in muscles and tissues of the body to facilitate a painless, why, blissful child birth. This flexibility is also is a logical extension of strength and endurance and hence "right nutrition". Fletcherism is all about "right nutrition" and that should say it all. It should take care of all the throwing ups, weight and health issues during pregnancy.

If Fletcherising can take the muscles and tissues of Fletcher and many others to the surprising levels of strength and endurance demonstrated by them even in old age, it can very well lead a mother's body to the peak of its strength, endurance and flexibility, making the most important and life giving experience of her life truly magical and blissful in every sense!

It's not that Fletcherism alone does it for you though. There are women who do not Fletcherise and still experience wonderful pregnancy with all the ease imaginable and later a blissful child birth. The most important factor here is the state of your mind, your thinking, and your feelings about the whole experience. Whatever age an expectant mum might be, and whatever complications others and she herself might see in her pregnancy or child birth, Fletcherising will help, in all cases, by all means. Knowing that you are doing the right thing for the both of you itself is a big morale booster.

Every moment is the perfect moment to take a good decision. You may be in your First, Second or your Third Trimester, or maybe even through with the trimesters and just awaiting the big day, there is no time as perfect as now to choose to eat well, to Fletcherise. It's like the X+ years of life discussed earlier that Fletcherism can give. If with the previous eating habits the level of discomfort would have been at a 5 on a scale of 1 to 10 (1 being the least and 10 being the most), Fletcherising can help reduce it to at least a 4. This is commendable progress nevertheless.

Here again, I am not suggesting that an expectant mum experiments with her diets, skips meals or ignores the advice of her doctors to rely purely on her own natural instincts and body signs. This may not work very well and may cause harm, reason being we lack practice and experience so do not want to be skipping our regular meal times waiting for true hunger to show up or suddenly throw away all the dietician prescribed diet charts and give in to our cravings. It's only with some practice and patient observation that one can differentiate between the habitual cravings and the true hunger. And this is not the time to experiment. There is only this one thing though that can be done, which cannot be harmful by any stretch of imagination, the main aspect of Fletcherising–chewing, munching, masticating as much as you can, whatever it is that has been prescribed for your diet—just masticate and see how it feels, right from the very first day!

So for all those expectant mums out there, Fletcherising could be one of the best choices you make for yourself, your loved ones who wish to see you comfortable and at ease during these days, and for that wonderful new life arriving into this world.

7

Transformed life

Anything which transforms our spiritual, mental or emotional realm does not leave the physical realm untouched. Almost all forms of Meditation have been proven to have a positive impact not only on mind but also on body, not just in the longer run but also sooner. In that case anything which has a profound impact on our physical realm would not leave the spiritual, mental or emotional realm untouched. Very few practices or routines be it exercise or diet or some other physical activity, have the level and depth of impact on our body as Fletcherism has. Fletcherism transforms our physical realm and so will essentially transform our spiritual, mental and emotional realm.

You don't have to try to make these changes happen, this transformation happens, you just need to sincerely Fletcherise and everything else will show up as obviously as weight loss does.

Mind Body: One big Whole

Listening to the body

"Listening to one's body" as Fletcherism calls for, can often be misinterpreted. Some may argue that it is because of listening to the body that they are sick in the first place, that's why they have been overeating always, craved always and so are overweight or unhealthy. It's always been about satisfying the needs of the body and hence the sorry state of affairs they are in. "Chewing" on this a little, it is quite apparent that the body has always given very physical signs indicating the nutritional abuse that is taking place. It has always cried out in a loud and clear voice that it is not happy with all that is being put into it. The signs such as loose motions, throwing ups, the heaviness after meals, the laziness, constipation, gases in stomach, acidity, excess weight gain, that tired feeling have all been the body's cry for help.

It's not the food or the drink causing this as we have seen, they cannot do any harm on their own. So if it's not the food or drink and not the body, it has to be the undisciplined mind which is the cause. Mind is cause of all trouble and Fletcherising addresses this in the most physical way.

Territory of mind

For many, the territory of mind is an un-ventured territory. Controlling directly, the urges of mind and its unstable characteristics is a Herculean task not everyone will be happy undertaking. The study of mind has gained a great momentum these days and many of us have joined in. But we also know how tough it is at times to keep on. Any "push" given to the mind is only met with an equal and opposite push (Newton's law).

Fletcherising is kind of a back door entry into the minds terrain. The mind would not notice immediately what Fletcherising can do to it and so will not resist it. The mind is busy enjoying the taste of the food while Fletcherising is working its magic on the body and on the ignorant mind. The mind unknowingly gets disciplined in its ways. It starts to love the body, it ceases to be the rebel it was and becomes caring and compassionate towards the house it stays in—this physical body. This explains why, by Fletcherising, one can overcome cravings and addictions with almost no resistance from the body or the mind.

One Body–One Mind–Lessons Learnt

Even though it seems most of the times that there are 10 different voices in our head and so maybe a number of minds, we nevertheless have only one mind. If it is disciplined in one area–Fletcherising, it becomes a habit with it, it will use this habit, the lessons learnt here, in rest of its businesses.

We all know in theory a number of good things and keep reading and reiterating these as well. But what we lack is experience. A thousand theories may be offered to prove something but till we experience it in our own minds and bodies, it remains theory with little or no practical value. As the saying goes, "an ounce of experience is worth a ton of theory", experience has a bigger impact on mind than theory! I have experienced a number of theories proved within a short period of Fletcherising. These lessons have been engraved deeply on my mind. This shows up not just when I am eating but also in other areas of my life because all said and done its one mind–one body and both have profound influences on each other.

I have always known theoretically that my body is the Temple of the Living God, that's what all the spiritual books say and I believed it to be true. As much as I wanted to do something which proved this, I never treated my body as a temple. If I was in charge of a real stone and cement Temple or Church or Mosque, I would not dump a truck load of garbage into these sacred places, I would not ignore their repair and maintenance requirements, I would not let germs and viruses prosper in there. I would keep it clean and sacred. This was not the way, not even close, to the way I was treating my body. I lived to eat remember! But with Fletcherism, I experience my physical self in a whole new way. The way I now treat my body makes me a proud caretaker of this beautiful Temple!

I always wanted empathy and selfless service to be a part of my personality, but it never was. I was sympathetic but not very empathetic. I have had my bit of struggle with weight loss and health issues like the many who continue to struggle with these. Since I was always so very self centered I never took notice of those around me struggling with the same issues and I had mine to solve anyways. But now since I have solved mine, I have this urge to reach out and help all those around me. Maybe it's just that I am noticing only now, there are so many out there who could do with some help. I see very few people

51

who probably look fit and healthy with a toned up body, tucked in tummy, a gait in their strides and so on–the physical signs of good health. A quick chat with them though reveals that majority of them force themselves to diets and exercise routines which, if they had some other option, they would never adopt. My heart seems to be reaching out to all of them, the way it never has, I have never been very high on my "Compassion quotient", but it seems to be going up now. And since its one mind-one body, compassion and empathy are becoming a part of my personality.

As noted earlier, a mind which is trained to be disciplined when eating, with regard to eating, adopts the discipline as a way of life eventually. One who is mindful of his ways of eating becomes mindful of the way he lives his life. A Fletcherite knows that there is only so much she can eat and so cannot dump anything and everything into her mouth and her stomach. She therefore learns to prioritize well in terms of what it is that she needs to eat. The priority setting skills are toned up and since it is a one Mind set up, this shows in every area of her life. Try it for yourself, become a Fletcherite and see how priority setting becomes easier than it was ever before. Be it at work, at home, with your social appointments, any area of your life–you will choose, you will prioritize, without hesitation, without regret or second thoughts. Life becomes a lot easier!

You will notice you are more focused than you previously were, with any task in hand. It's again the one mind principle. If your mind knows now to focus on the taste of the food in the mouth and how to stay present, it will start being present more often. Even if you are used to watching Television while eating (like I was), this habit will change automatically. You will find that there is nothing more enjoyable in that moment when you are eating, than the taste of the food. Eating kind of becomes a very sacred, focused and enjoyable ceremony.

This internal transformation takes place in bits and pieces and without you actually realizing it is taking place. That's why it is faced with least or no resistance from any part of you–mind or body. And when the mind and body are synchronized in their efforts and goals, there is no stopping them–it's a double team and will not stop till the goal of a complete transformation is achieved!

Physical Changes Other Than Eating Habits

Some other physical areas of transformation you may notice in yourself could be your body posture, in the way you walk, in the way you breathe–your body posture will get more straight, weather you are walking or sitting. Your shoulders will get pulled back, chest out, stomach in. This happens as soon as you get close to your perfect weight. The stretched and straight body posture opens up the space inside the chest; the lungs seem to get expanded easily to allow deep breathing. You don't consciously do it, you start realizing that something is changing, you start realizing that in the way you walked and breathed all your life till now, something is not right, you may start experiencing some pain here and there and then all of a sudden, you realize intuitively what needs changing. You just straighten up one fine day! There would be kind of gait in your strides replacing the drag which may have been the norm.

As strange as it may sound, your lifelong habit of using a pillow when sleeping might be gone suddenly, it may just disappear a few months into Fletcherising. You may start sleeping straight on your back even though you were used to sleeping sideways since childhood. I was surprised when this happened. I was happy to learn later that the best position for sleeping is on your back without a pillow. This enables the spine to rest fully, straight, soothing the aches or pains if any from a day full of activity and business. This position prevents neck pain, enables deep breathing. Some doctors do believe sleeping on your back without a pillow is the best sleeping position though not much research has gone into it to prove it. Here again Nature has not left us without help, the design of our body suggests the spine and upwards to the neck and head were created to remain straight. Nature did know we will need to sleep, but it did not give us an inward curve on the back of our necks to accommodate a pillow. So I choose to believe that this change in sleeping habits I experienced cannot be a coincidence in that case. Every process in the body seems to have started aligning itself with the Natures "Perfect way". It's the one body-one mind principle again!

All these changes are what I started experiencing a few months into Fletcherising. There are many more surprises in store for me I know which will be revealed as I walk this path.

This holds true for every Fletcherite. Because no two bodies are alike, these changes will occur but within different timeframes. For some it may be sooner than it was for me and for some it may be later. But it will come as a natural transition.

Freedom from Addictions and Cravings

In his books Horace Fletcher has given several illustrations of alcoholics turning sober because of Fletcherising. One cannot get high on alcohol if they Fletcherise every sip. It may be too much to ask of a person addicted to alcoholic drinks to Fletcherise his drinks. So they will not Fletcherise their drinks, never mind, they can do this with their food. Once they start Fletcherising their food, this habit of Fletcherising is contagious and will eventually flow over to their drinks as well. This is because for a Fletcherite, passing anything down the throat except for water, without Fletcherising, is a sin. This transition is unavoidable.

Fletchers experience with his own drinking habits and those of the ordinary Tramps picked up from the street of Chicago makes this amply clear, he notes,"…. *They (the tramps) simply ate what they chose to order from the bill of fare of a cheap restaurant, but were told to chew everything for all it was worth, which they made no objection to doing. Time was of no value to them, and they really discovered new delights of gustatory pleasure which they had not known before. My tramps were beery and bleary as tramps generally are, but not so dirty; for I paid for baths, washing, and in some instances furnished clothing. Besides supplying these luxuries, I gave them occasionally a big silver dollar which they called a ""cart wheel."" It was surprising to see these degenerates freshen up in appearance and lose their blotchiness and greasiness of facial appearance. I knew how to talk to them to get their confidence, and they looked on me as just another "freak" like themselves, but with some kind of a money "pull."*

Up to the time I began my own experiment, I had been a social drinker of alcohol in all forms to the full extent of "gentlemanly decency," with occasional slips when near the outer edge that made me ashamed of myself after I got sober again. Not only were social occasions an excuse, but I often ordered the social occasions to serve as an excuse.

The result of my own pursuit of thorough tasting of my food had been that my own ponderosity of front weight fell off, and at the same time I had no desire for wine or beer. It was all a surprise to me, but it was not an amazing surprise until one day one of my tramp guests came to me and said: "Boss, this eatin" game is great; think of me with a dollar in my pocket and not wantin" beer." In a short time I forgot that I had ever liked wine or beer. It never occurred to me to order it except for a guest, and then I took it with him, or, rather them, for there were usually several or many at my eating parties, but in the Fletcherian manner which is so eminently Epicurean that a few sips went as far as a half bottle used to do.

Fletcher had once demonstrated Fletcherism to the "one bottle" wine consumers. He guided them to Fletcherise Wine. They were doing it for the first time and yet had the very same experience as Fletcher had in the enjoyment of the wine and in responding to the natural appetite on the quantity of wine consumed. Half a bottle of wine gave them (a dozen or more members of the Club who participated in the experiment) more satisfaction than any of them knew was possible.

Fletcherising, even if it starts only with food, eventually inspires you to be responsible. One, you wouldn't put any un-Fletcherised food or drink into your body, so if its alcohol that is the addiction, that will be taken care of and two, you start caring about your body so much that you wouldn't even think of causing it any harm by putting in any harmful substance into it. It would be like what I experienced, you would treat your body as a Temple and keep it sacred and clean. This in turn will take care of smoking and drugs which technically cannot be Fletcherised but are harmful and polluting substances nevertheless. Once a Fletcherite you would never pollute your Body Temple!

This will be a natural and almost an unconscious transition again. You will not experience any résistance. You will protect yourself from all the harm (as you would protect your child) lovingly and there is this feeling of pride and happiness knowing you are taking care of yourself. This feeling gives you a bigger kick than any of the alcoholic drinks would. This is as an icing on the cake. It makes the self chosen (and not self-imposed) discipline worthwhile. It is but natural therefore for a person who has not even thought of giving up smoking or drinking, to give up these once he turns a Fletcherite with no internal or external force. There will be no feeling of sacrifice or deprivation, but just a sense of pride and happiness.

The de-addiction centers and programs help a great deal in overcoming addictions. Sometimes they take care of the problem permanently whereas many a times, the addict gets de-addicted only to go back to the addiction after a while sooner or later. The major reason for this failure is the fact that they force themselves to give up or deprive themselves of that which they are addicted to. There is this gravitational pull which is subsided for a while at the de addiction camp or during the de-addiction program but the fire is still burning within. The lack of will power adds oil to the fire and the addiction returns. Repeated failure in this venture sometimes disappoints and discourages the person so much that they simply give up on trying to give up the addiction. There is another important aspect which is the cause of these failures–the focus is on the "addiction", on smoking, on drinking, on drugs. For some it's like saying, "don't think about a pink elephant".

Fletcherising on the other hand does not force you to give up anything, the transition happens, but in the most natural and effortless way. The focus here is also not the "addiction".

Use of will power is required of course but if it is for something you are not attached to or do not crave for, it comes easily. For example if one has this craving to eat and has in front of her, her favorite food, the urge is strong and uncontrollable at times and she would need to really hold herself back using some mental force. But if the food in front of her is not one of her favorites, she may still eat it, but the urge will not be strong and she may be able to avoid it completely with a fairly lesser degree of mental force. So an addict can start Fletcherising something that is easy to Fletcherise. So yes, Fletcherising can start with food alone at first and the transition will take place naturally –remember the Tramp who said,: ***"Boss, this eatin" game is great; think of me with a dollar in my pocket and not wantin" beer."*** Once a Fletcherite, always a Fletcherite, Fletcherite in one area cannot *not* be a Fletcherite in another!

It is not intended to advise that if a person is undergoing a treatment for de-addiction, it be stopped with a sole reliance on Fletcherism. Fletcherism works but the person may lack practice and may harm herself in the process for want of some external guidance. The willingness to "chew your drinks and drink your food" is all that is needed to get started, rest will be taken care of by Nature.

Our Belief Systems and the Law of Attraction

I have attended several courses for self-development, read several books on Law of Attraction, attended tele seminars and webinars. They all have life changing power–they are all what they claim to be–Transformational tools. Tools that can change my life, change the way I feel, make me a happier, healthier and more peaceful me. Their content and delivery keeps up the promise in every sense. And I have benefited greatly from these programs, just that manifestation of my desires, health, wealth, happiness, did not seem as easy as it should have been. These programs touch mind and through which we try to change "matter"–health and wealth for e.g. The road block I met with was the fact that for me and my senses, I am "matter" first and then "mind". That is even if I believe with all my heart and mind that I am a spiritual being having a physical experience, I still seem to have trouble experiencing it that way. The stress of the daily routine life seems to get the best of me making me realize I am very much physical. So the fact remains that even though while we continue to work on our minds to accept the fact and reality that we are actually spiritual beings, we need to do something for the "matter"–our bodies and finances as well.

This may not be true for some who are really powerful with their belief systems and can make miracles happen, but for me, I have not yet developed enough powers to instantly manifest my health goals for e.g.–strength, endurance and radiant health through imagination and affirmations only. The "Belief" that by changing my beliefs around the topic of heath, by affirming a thousand times that I am healthy, I am going to become healthy, did not work fully for me. I did feel far better than I used to, but taking an example of my weight, it wasn't reducing on its own without me taking any efforts. Efforts in the form of exercising or diet control which was not something I enjoyed doing. The process of manifestation had to be an "inspired action" as Law of Attraction says, it should not feel anything but good, it should be a WIN WIN! My affirmations and visualizations did not reduce my weight, but they sure did bring me to Fletcherism–I get to eat all that I love, I do not force myself to exercise, I lost weight, I am gaining health–it's a WIN WIN!

This ounce of experience of Law of Attraction for me is worth more than all the theory I have read on this subject. My mind has experienced that the Law of Attraction works. It knows that we–mind and body, together has made it possible and that the power of manifestation indeed is in my own hands.

What is happening now as a result of this "experienced belief" is I am leading a healthy lifestyle, I am living my dream of coaching and counseling people on this healthy life style, I am living my dream of writing a book, of becoming a published Author, of sharing my experience with the world, of doing my bit for the health and well being of the entire human race!

It worked for me this way, it may work for you in some other way. Nature, Universe, Creator are all the different names of that one source which is all knowing, which is a sum total of all the laws, Law of attraction being one of them. The physical evidence which a manifested desire offers convinces you of your power to create your own reality. Like me there may be several who wish to be back to the weight they were while in their college days, or maybe you are in college or school and wish to get fit, the first step of which is losing weight if you are overweight and gaining weight if you are underweight. When you experience this manifestation in such a natural way, as a result of your own conscious choices, your mind knowingly or unknowingly gets convinced of your power of creation, of the existence of the "perfect way" in everything. And when you unlock the "perfect way" within even one of the Natures processes, the others seem to follow–that's Law of Attraction at work. You start finding "perfect ways" out of any and every situation, any problem, you find the "perfect way" of life. It's very easy when you start walking on the Natures way, you automatically follow the Natures laws, even if you do not consciously realize that you are. Everything that you encounter on this natural route will be nothing but natural and "natural" is always "magical"!

Economical benefits

Fletcher was invited once for a meal and this is what he observed when they finished the meal: "*Both my host and my hostess declared that they had never enjoyed a summer evening meal more, and yet all that was ordered was not consumed, while the cost, for the three, was less than a dollar for the food alone. The method employed to interpret appetite (ordering what first comes to mind and then stop–baked potatoes and green corn) was a revelation to my friends. They were accustomed to ordering several courses for each person, although they thought they were "small eaters" and economic feeders. Had they ordered for us three without my assistance, the dinner would not have cost less than four or five dollars, and with a plethora of food on the table all would have felt it necessary to eat as much as possible, in order to get value received.*"

There is another story when a Fletcherite friend of Fletcher went to lunch with a generous host in New York, and the following conversation about the lunch to be ordered was heard, "*What will you have? What! Only a baked potato and a bottle of ginger ale? All right for a starter; but what are you really going to have? Nothing more! What is the matter with you? Come, now; tell me what you want for lunch? Stocks are badly off, but I haven't reached the starvation point yet. Don't treat me like* that when I'm trying to treat you right and white. Brace up, old man, and have something to eat." The intermediate replies can be imagined as in an overheard telephone conversation.

The result of a group of missionary workers teaching Fletcherism is also a fascinating example; "*More than a thousand persons were saving an average of $3.00 a month on the cost of their sustenance, and were temperance converts through the sloughing off of all desire for their moonshine product (cheap whisky). Think of a saving from sheer waste of $3,000 a month ($36,000 a year) to a community where $1,000 is considered to be a princely fortune, and a saving of a thousand human units from the scrap-heap of worse than death!*"

In my own experience, my usual spending on food has come down by 50% since the quantity I was used to eating has also come down to about 50% now. It's when I eat out with family or friends that I notice the economical benefits all the more. I was amongst the biggest contributors to the total expenditure and now it seems I am the smallest. The total bill of eating out has been cut down. I don't feel the need to order a separate dish for myself anymore and fortunately since I love all types of food, I manage to find something my appetite craves for but which is in the plates of my friends or family. I seem to get a wider variety than the rest since I pick a bite or two from every dish and since the quantity I pick is so small, no one seems to mind!

If yours is a Fletcherites' family, your households monthly expenditure will be cut down by about 50%, which is a very good saving indeed.

Fletcherising therefore also improves your finances–the very important tool which in the modern and inflation ridden world today is of paramount importance.

Know Thyself

"KNOW THYSELF" is one of the chapters in "The New Glutton or Epicure" which says,

"Know Thyself" has been the admonition of sages from earliest times. "Become acquainted with our Normal Instincts, with Appetite and with our food chemist, Taste and follow their directions with implicit confidence", is the admonition taught by our experiments, for they can lead you to robust health and greatly increased vigor of the body and mind. Study and heed them patiently for a week and you will follow their invitations and warnings through life.

Thorough repair of an impaired body may not be effected immediately, although wonderful results—almost miraculous—have been attained in three months; but a week's faithful and attentive study of the possibilities of Epicureanism, with right alimentation as its basic requirement, in adding to the comfort and enjoyment of life will result in right eating being made philosophically and religiously habitual, and will give a backbone of Epicurean character that will not easily succumb to gluttonous impetuosity.

*The more we learn, the more evident it is that there is a **Perfect Way** locked, or rather, enfolded, in all of Nature's secrets, and that it is intended that man shall sometime discover them."*

There are wealth, health, strength, long life abundant usefulness and much resultant happiness offered as a reward for learning and following Nature's Perfect Way."

Those with some serious health issues and under medication or prescribed diet probably may not and should not be very adventurous by ignoring the external medical help and relying solely on their own natural instincts. But those who are "technically" fit and healthy can give Fletcherising a fair try, in its entirety by being patient and listening to what the Nature is telling us. There is this tendency with most of us to take outside help—doctors, medicines, pills, as soon as we notice even the slightest of disharmony in any part of our being. For those with serious ailments, it's understandable. But the technically "fit" ones also seem to do the same. We all seem to trust everyone else more than we trust ourselves. It's like saying your friends, family, doctors know you better than you know yourself. Is it true? I guess not, if not, then of course you know yourself the best. So you are the one who knows and should be advising yourself on what and how much you need to eat at any given point of time. The gyms and dieticians are doing a great job else what would the majority of us who have not yet started trusting self do? We would be so miserable without their help. They are a blessing indeed while we are still learning to trust ourselves.

No two bodies are alike and so no two eating requirements are alike. Who other than you knows you the best? Why not give yourself the chance then to decide your own good at least for a week to begin with. This one week can then be transformed to a lifetime not by force but by conscious willing choice!

Fletcher notes, "*Nature cannot be profitably studied alone through books. Nature has a separate message for each intelligence. Each body machine has peculiarities which the possessor alone can understand. Object lessons, personally experienced or observed, are the best. "Once seeing (or feeling) is worth a hundred times telling about," is a wise Japanese proverb; and it is true.*"

Fletcherising helps you train yourself to be a good listener, a good observer, it helps you know yourself. Fletcherise and you will experience Nature first hand, know yourself truly, in the real sense, maybe for the first time since you thought you knew yourself!

8

Fletcherism–Making it a Habit

This Fletcherising business may sound like a very strenuous and cumbersome task. But believe me when I say this, it's just a matter of getting into the habit of Fletcherising and then when the results start showing, they will be worth much more than the efforts. It's a one stop shop for all the health needs and comes with a life time guarantee.

Some may wish to embrace this theory and practice in its entirety, paying attention to every aspect–the When, What, How and How much–for both food and drinks. There are many who can muster up their will power, or already have the level of will power, to start all at once, completely leaving behind the old eating habits and adopt Fletcherism as the new way of eating from the very first day. They may not mind skipping a couple of meals, giving up on the habits of eating between meals and waiting patiently to see how a true and earned appetite feels. They may also be able to focus on the taste, observe the various processes that go on in the mouth, the food touching the tongue, the secretion of saliva, the grinding of the teeth, the closing and opening of food filter, the involuntary swallowing etc. i.e. following all the Five Principles of Fletcherism as discussed in the opening of the first chapter. This is possible and not very difficult to achieve. It does need a level of control though and will power which may be a challenge for some. Even for those who take up this challenge, it may seem like a bit of a drag initially to pay attention to all the aspects and in this the main thing, the taste kind of gets ignored. As a result the enjoyment disappears for a while. It's like learning to drive. It is such a conscious and focused effort in the beginning, you have to remember to use the clutch and the brake appropriately, change the gears based on your speed level, when to slow down, when to speed up, looking in the rear view mirror and so on. In all of this one important element goes missing–the pleasure of driving. It is the same with Fletcherising, but this is easier than driving as there is only one thing that needs focus, the taste. Everything else falls into place. Yes cravings may show up and you may binge but not as much as you used to, so binge if you must, but still, chew.

Whether or not someone goes fast track or goes slow and steady depends on how desperate he or she is to see the visible, provable solution to their health problems, to do the one right thing and rest easy!

As for me–This was my best and the last shot after all the partially and temporarily successful experiments with diets and exercising. I had pinned all my hopes on Fletcherism and so was kind of desperate on finding out if this indeed works. It did work, so I did hit the Bulls Eye with this one but made a few mistakes which threw cold water on my efforts once in a while. I have had set backs and have fallen down and gotten up again. It's discouraging and disappointing at times to fall down when you are running compared to when you are walking. It's good sometimes to go slow and progress steadily rather than to go fast, fall and then get up. This is especially for those who have the tendency to give up quickly, writing it off as "it doesn't work". However once you start seeing the results–the feeling in your stomach and the visible change in your body, weather you are running or walking, you will want to keep going even if there are lapses and moments of cravings which make you give in.

In this process of failing and getting up again, I have learnt a lot of lessons. Had I known these earlier, I could have avoided them and would have made this journey all the more pleasurable. I would have progressed and moved only forward.

Deciding to Fletcherise is a very important initiative, probably the best thing you could do for the health of your physical body to begin with. The best thing you can do for your mind is feeding it constantly with good positive thoughts. Likewise, the best thing you can do for your body is feeding it the right nutrition, Fletcherised food! If you wish to take this path, there are a few things to be kept in mind, in order to give this initiative a long life and to make it self-sustaining. These may look too small to warrant a mention and because of this very reason, get ignored.

Slow and Steady if you wish to

Day and time

Why choose a particular day and time? It is because you don't want to be sabotaging yourself on day one, you don't want to stop even before you start. It makes a lot of difference if you get a good start. For people like me who are used to sabotaging every new initiative, a successful start is of paramount importance. It's like "well begun is work half done". Try and succeed the first time you do it and you want to have another date with Fletcherism. And so a day when your "Acceptance of a new idea quotient" is at its peak would be good, so it may not be a Monday morning for some. The day when you think you may have some time is when you can start, not when you are in a hurry to finish off the meal. Start Fletcherising at a time when you are not very hungry starving or craving, as you may not be very patient to be patiently munching the bites you are taking and may gulp it down as usual to fill up the *perceived* vacuum in the stomach. Having said that, the best day is always **today a**nd the best time is always **now.**

Start small

Any change causes initial resistance, if this is big which talks about changing a lifetime of habits, it may cause resistance for some–the opposing force of old habits. Things slow down even before they pick up speed.

Instead of deciding that you will Fletcherise every meal every day for rest of your life, it would be good to say to yourself that today for the first 5 minutes of my meal time in the afternoon / evening, I will Fletcherise. Whatever it is that I am eating, for the first 5 minutes, I will Fletcherise. I will let nothing other than thoroughly masticated food pass down my throat for these first 5 minutes. If you go in a group for lunch and don't want to be trying it out in front of others, 5 minutes before you leave for lunch, take a bite of anything you may have with you, a biscuit, a chocolate, a piece of cake—Fletcherise for 5 minutes today if you can, yes you can if you will! This works even for the biggest of self-sabotagers!

Once you have done your 5 minutes today, which is a success, small but still a success, it encourages you to take the next step forward. Decide that the for the next 2 days or a week you will do it—5 minutes of Fletcherising at any one meal time, not necessarily breakfast or dinner or lunch. Feel free to increase it to 10 or 15 minutes based on your comfort zone. When you touch the 15 minute Fletcherising mark, you may be surprised to note that your appetite may already have been satisfied. That is you are no longer hungry for the time being, and you may decide you don't need any more food for the moment. Fletcherising does this. Once you know "How to eat" the "When, What and How Much" eventually falls in place, sooner than later.

Initial trials—make it exciting

Make these initial trials as exciting as possible. Decide to Fletcherise for 5 minutes, your favorite chocolate, crisps, coffee, a piece of your favorite cake, ice cream, anything that you love to eat or drink. Get all the taste that you can out of it. Don't bother about swallowing, just let it melt into your mouth, grind it with your teeth, roll it around in your mouth with your tongue. Taste every bit of that piece of chocolate, that bite of cake, enjoy it for all its worth. This will give you a feel of how Fletcherising feels, it feels delicious!

Here again, with Freedom comes Responsibility (discussed in more detail later). The start needs to be as exciting as possible but not too exciting with only chocolates and cakes being eaten for couple of meals on couple of days for that matter. That could be the habitual craving and not the calling of natural appetite. So yes you are free, but you need to be responsible.

21 days

Most of us have heard or read that it takes 21 repetitions to make it a habit. That is to consciously form a habit or move away from a bad habit, you have to stick to your resolve for 21 days at a stretch. Thereafter it stays alive drawing its strength from the basic framework of human behavior, human mind which is designed to feed and keep habits alive.

Once you are successful in meeting your predetermined target of 5 /10 /15 minutes of Fletcherising for a week, decide now to do it for 3 weeks 21 days or 30 days if possible—one whole month! Just one meal per day Fletcherised for 5 /10 / 15 minutes. It is quite possible that by the time you finish your 30 days, you might have turned a complete Fletcherite. Fletcherising will have become a habit by then and would have spilled over into all the meals you have at different times of the day. If the resolve to Fletcherise is maintained for 21 days, 3 weeks that is, it is enough to change the old eating habits. Why 21 days, as advised by Fletcher even a week of sincere and fully dedicated observation and action can do it for you, for those who *will*. And this is true, even though it may take time for some to get the "When, What and How Much" right, most will find that even after only a week of Fletcherising, the "How" replaces the old gulping down habits. I found it very difficult, rather impossible to go back to my old "non-chewing habits" after only a week. And this is enough to keep you going.

It may not be a coincidence that the easiest bit is the "How". This is the most delicious bit. One may find it difficult to capture the signs from within which say the "When, What and How much" initially but "How" couldn't have been easier, you know it from the very first day! Nature couldn't have made it easier than this for us. The Creators designs and plans are marvelous. We just need to keep munching on the amazing taste that the food offers and slowly but eventually the other aspects will be set right. One thing that would need to speed up is the movement of the jaws. This raises the taste quotient, increases the secretion of saliva and gets the best out of the food quicker.

Meals and drinks when short on time:

I used to drink a big full cup of milk every morning before I went to work. I used to drink it like water. I loved it alright but never really tasted it as much as I do now. It now takes at least 15 to 20 minutes for me to Fletcherise and finish off the usual quantity I used to drink. I don't have so much of time to spare in the morning, so I take a bottle of milk to work. I sip at it when I feel like and taste it for all its worth before it disappears into my mouth and down the throat, involuntarily.

The fact remains that I cannot now drink that quantity I used to, all at once. I drink it in intervals over a time frame of 4 to 6 hours. Maybe I don't need to carry on drinking so much of milk, but I love it and am not going to give it up voluntarily. If it's not required by my body, I will eventually give it up, but involuntarily.

This applies to the breakfast, lunch or any other meal you wish to have but are short of time. It's much better to skip a meal than to eat in a hurry. And missing meals is not going to do you any harm but eating in a hurry and not Fletcherising will definitely do.

Keeping the plate least loaded

Do not decide at the very beginning of the meal as to the quantity you would be eating. If you are used to taking 4 loafs of bread into your plate before you start eating, try taking one first. After you finish that, take another and if you still have any appetite left take the third or anything else your appetite wishes to have. Putting more into the plate often creates a kind of subconscious pressure on the mind, the pressure to finish all that is taken. This discourages Fletcherising as we start wondering how much time it would take to finish all this with the pace with which we are eating.

Likewise when we see a table full of a variety of our favorite food laid out, especially when we are out on parties, we tend to take a lot on our plate falling prey to our habitual cravings and assuming that we are going to eat all that, and we actually end up eating all that to avoid "food wastage". Fletcher says select that which most appeals to your appetite, take a small quantity, Fletcherise and then check if you need more of it or do you need anything else instead. Have all you want, slow and steady, Fletcherise! Have to mention here, this habit is carried forward in other areas of life as well. If you are used to having your plate full all the time, things are surely going to change.

Next bite waiting

Most of us have this habit of putting a morsel of food into our mouth and before we finish chewing and swallowing that, keeping another morsel ready on the tip of the fork and on the way to our mouths. This again creates a kind of subconscious pressure on the entire machinery of ours which then tries to push a job half done (un-chewed food), into the next process (digestion). Under a pressure like this, mouth tries to swallow what's in there as soon as it can and the hand which is holding the second morsel comes in as fast as it can. We don't want to be causing undue pressure on our digestive apparatus. So what we can do is once we take a bite, keep down whatever that is we are taking a bite from, cross our hands, clasp our hands, do anything but touch the second morsel till the first one has been Fletcherised and involuntary swallowed.

The table manners

When there are the fibrous remains of chicken, fish or meat in your mouth and there comes this time to remove it from your mouth in a party, when you are on the table with friends, business partners, colleagues, don't worry too much about table manners. You can pretend to be wiping your mouth with a tissue and remove remains into the tissue if taking it out with hand bothers you. Trust me, it doesn't feel the least bit embarrassing. You feel quite funny actually and childlike too when you do this, you smile at yourself, you simply adore the innocent beautiful you in that moment when you are so caring, considerate and sensitive to you!

Discuss

Talk about Fletcherising to your loved ones. When you talk more about it the understanding of the theory of Fletcherism starts sinking in. This aids the ultimate practice. I have started paying more attention to Fletcherising and have been doing it better since I started advising those who asked, and more so since I started writing this book. Talk about it as much as you can, but make sure you talk to those who are interested and won't discourage you. We don't want to be discouraged if not encouraged.

Making it a habit

It is better to cultivate this habit for once and reap the benefits of a life time. If I was offered a lifetime solution to a problem which requires me to spend one month of constant awareness and hard work, it's a small price to pay. Its rather not a price at all, you will be reaping the benefits right during the process as well, your benefit is all the taste you taste like never before. One month of sincere efforts, you see the results, not just feel it (you start feeling the difference even after one week into it). Weight loss is the first sign (weight gain if you are underweight). You automatically get motivated to carry on further thus making it a habit. Imagine if you were brought up with this eating habit, would you find it difficult? No, it just takes some persistence and patience to carry on like this and then it becomes a habit and man (read that woman as well) is a creature of habits. So Fletcherism is not difficult at all, it's only the willingness of making it a habit that requires some work.

Some more words of inspiration–habit in a day!

The story of Fletchers friend should add to the inspiration here: This is Fletchers friend to Fletcher (from The New Glutton or Epicure): *"You remember the state of health I was in when we met here in the Waldorf five years ago. If I hadn't been struck by the marvelous alteration in your appearance from what it was when I had seen you last, I should have been terribly bored by your relation of your experience, for I was sick to death of mention of cures and diet-regimens of all sorts. But you astonished me so by your changed appearance, and I was in such a hopeless condition, that I thought I would give your scheme a trial. Next day my breakfast, which was also my lunch, for I was feeling too badly to get up earlier, brought me some sweet corn as one of the several items I habitually ordered. In giving this corn thorough chewing before swallowing, I noticed that, while the inside of the corn liquefied readily and was quickly swallowed, there remained in my mouth a collection of the hulls, and these invited the bad table manners of "spitting out". I removed this collection of refuse, and, on examination, found that it consisted of hard substance that I never had noticed before in connection with cooked sweet corn. This set me to thinking. What had I not been putting into my stomach all these years in my ignorance of the constituents of this one kind of common food, and what not in other foods that I had not yet observed?*

In continuing the observation further, I discovered that many of the foods that I was accustomed to take contained hard, insoluble ingredients or cottony fiber that got more and more cottony and refractory with mastication. In trying coffee, my favorite beverage, as you told me I might do if I handled it rightly in the mouth, I tasted it until it was absorbed or swallowed involuntarily just as you told me the expert wine tasters and tea tasters do. I sipped and enjoyed my small cup of coffee as I had never done before in my life, and knew afterwards that it had not hurt me as usual, as no immediate protest came from the stomach, which formerly had been the case. I slept the "sleep of the just" that night, and awoke in fine form next morning. From that day to this I have not been troubled with indigestion, and during these five years I have not been sick a day or an hour or a moment, and have slept like a babe."

This change was not over months or years, the habit was developed by Fletchers friend in a day! This is not difficult at all as you don't have to give up anything or change anything. It's just that whatever time you have set aside for your meals, Fletcherise and eat as much as you can in that time. If that means you have eaten only half the quantity you usually would have eaten, be it so. Actually it is just right, just enough for now. Wait until hunger shows up next.

Yes it may take a while, but since you are starting small, the resistance is the least, it eventually creeps in like a habit and getting rid of a habit is not an easy task.

Some Misconceptions, Pitfalls and Workarounds

Because we are so used to relying on our doctors, dieticians, physical trainers, and trusting everything that is complicated, it becomes difficult to rely on our own guidance; we doubt the simplicity of the process and question its results. Even when we start experiencing the benefits, there is a degree of skepticism in it and a feeling that something could be going wrong because we are on our own here. But we are not on our own here, Horace Fletcher and several others have walked this path prescribed by Nature and have reaped nothing but benefits. Having said that, it is quite easy to fall prey to the doubts and worries which come with a lack of confidence in self, lack of confidence in the fact that *you* know yourself the best and not *those others* who think you are wrong. There are some misconceptions about Fletcherism which I have come across whenever I mentioned Fletcherism to anyone. There are also some pitfalls created by our own belief systems that can be easily avoided.

Fletcherism is not about eating less or starving yourself:

The quantity of food I eat is fairly little and when people see how much I eat, they immediately dismiss the idea of Fletcherising saying they cannot eat so less. They need to eat more to be strong. They also think that I am losing weight because I am starving myself and so I am weak and undernourished. What they don't understand is that you don't have to force yourself to give up half the quantity of food you previously eat. You just have to allow the natural transition to take place. Eat as much as your body allows you to. Yes the body will require less now because the food is in such a digestion friendly and nutritious state when it goes into your body that there is lesser wastage and the body finds it enough. So for all those who think they cannot survive with a lesser quantity of food, it's not about the quantity, it's about the quality (Fletcherised food) which will automatically lead you to a lower quantity with absolutely no feeling of deprivation or losing of strength. Eat as much as you can, but Fletcherise.

Skipping meals–caution

When I started Fletcherising I did not go slow and steady, I went Fast Track, a bit too fast probably. So much so that in the first week I skipped quite some meals and completely stopped having my breakfast to find out how "true hunger" felt. I didn't feel true hunger, but I did feel a surge in the gases in my stomach (which was used to being full and now suddenly it was all empty, it caught air it seemed). I felt a bit weak with all the starving. Horace Fletcher says that once you start Fletcherising even if you skip meals for longer periods, you will not feel weak, rather you are not supposed to be feeling weak or having headaches if you don't eat for couple of days since we have the Ten Horse power capacity within us all the time, just that we don't know it. But I agree that's not the experience most of us have had. So in the initial days, it is advisable to pay attention to how you feel about this whole thing. I stopped having my breakfast completely later on and after a couple of months of Fletcherising, tried skipping all meals for 2 days as an experiment to see how it feels, it surprisingly felt okay. I didn't feel weak or tired because of the lack of food. I have my breakfast now when I am hungry, I don't if I am not.

If you are okay skipping meals since you do not know the true hunger do it, or simply to test your endurance, do it if you want to, else it's good to continue with your usual meals but only chewing more, as much as you can.

Those with some ailments that require taking of medicines at regular intervals–after /before meals etc, or those on specific prescribed diets / exercise routines are advised not to be very adventurous with skipping meals. There is nothing like "excess Fletcherising" or "drawbacks of Fletcherising" for anyone, even for those with serious ailments, but relying on self alone in the beginning when you lack the practice or experience is what may cause harm.

Right focus–taste

The food may lose its taste completely if the concentration is only on chewing. No taste would mean no saliva. Its painfully boring to try and force the secretion of saliva when you are concentrating on chewing alone and not on taste. When the concentration is on the taste, chewing and secretion of saliva are effortless. Secretion of Saliva is greatly reduced if the thoughts are not on the food being eaten. For e.g. watching television, talking, thinking about the next course–these things you will notice slow down the secretion of saliva. Complete focus on the meal ensures plentiful secretion of saliva and brings out the taste most deliciously. Initially it may seem like too much of efforts to concentrate on food alone especially if you are used to watching television, reading newspaper etc. during meals. But once you start enjoying the process, the focus will be the food; the focus will be the taste!

Confusion–internal conflict

Sometimes you see your favorite food in front of you, one which you have been helping yourself to for about 2 or three plateful of servings, and now your habit wants you to do the same but you will not be able to. This happens when you are a few days into Fletcherising. There is this internal conflict going on, which previously would end up in you binging and then feeling guilty, but now ends up in you restraining yourself reluctantly maybe, but fairly effortlessly and later blessing yourself for doing so. Instead of getting irritated with this conflict it's good to notice that you are marching forward. This is indeed one big step forward.

Sudden weight loss–and "words of discouragement"

Sudden weight loss is usually seen as a sign of a disease or some ill health. It's strange why it is not associated with an improvement of health first. As for me when I went on a rapid weight loss spree, I did look a bit tired and sick because of all the excess starving I did in the first week, but later on as well when I started eating well, the weight loss was inevitable. Number of people wanted to know how I lost 30 pounds in 15 weeks and an equal number of people thought and took the liberty of asking me if I was sick (or even telling me that I look sick) or have been seriously sick and thereby losing so much of weight. Family and friends were quite concerned since they thought I could be sick. This concern is understandable. It can be very discouraging and scary sometimes. If you are not careful, you may actually start feeling sick and worried about why you are losing so much of weight. Plus once you turn a Fletcherite, your food intake reduces to at least or sometimes even more than 50%, another reason for those who think you are sick to believe that yes you are sick and weak and that this is not a healthy weight loss, that you are starving yourself to lose weight. But this is not true. I did fall for this and for about a month or so struggled to convince myself and others that I was very much healthy. I fell sick once in the process with flu because I was quite convinced that I was weak and my immune system was also weak and so I can easily catch the flu that was making rounds in those days. I did catch it. I did not have to, but I did, but I also recovered from it sooner than others, and with a bare minimum of medicines, thereby restoring my faith in health, in Fletcherism.

I fell for the "words of discouragement". This reaction from onlookers is understandable because this surprisingly simple Health Mantra—Fletcherism is so surprisingly unpopular. You lose weight rapidly, head to toe, your wedding ring may fall off if you don't realize your fingers are slimmer now. An old shoe of yours may feel like it is one size bigger than your feet. The age old, stubborn belly fat melts away, the tummy gets tucked in. your buttocks, your arms, your thighs, every part of your body you have been struggling with for so long to lose weight, suddenly loses weight. You are not trying to work separately on your arms, your thighs, your buttocks, your waist, but still every part of your body which has had these stubborn layers of fat loses weight. This could be unheard of in your group, your social circle, but it is perfectly normal, good health and natural weight will follow Fletcherism.

Fine chubby people look cuter and sweeter compared to those who are just at the right weight. I was chubbier and looked really sweet as I get told nowadays and that I don't look that good anymore. But ask these chubby sweet people, ask me how I felt then, I never felt this good. It's not just about "looking fat" here, it's about the state of health risk you are in. A couple of months into Fletcherising I was told by some, that this was good enough and I should not lose more weight, to which my question was and is, there are only two things I am doing—eating right and a moderate level of activity—would you suggest I stop walking and moving around or I start eating anything and everything, anytime and every time like I used to in the past? Which of these two should I stop doing? They don't know what to answer. I cannot stop anything midway now, if my frame was not supposed to hold more than a 100 pounds (Nature assigned weight and not the "standard"), I may continue losing weight till I reach that point since there is a lot of dead stock, garbage that I am carrying inside. Once I get rid of all that I will retain a constant weight.

The last thing on my mind when I started was "looking good", I was after "feeling good" and "looking good" follows as an essential by product. But then be prepared for these words of discouragement in the meanwhile from those who are used to seeing you chubby and sweet!

Freedom and Responsibility

Fletcherism gave me the liberty to eat what I want, it released me from the need to force myself to exercise against my own will. "With great power, comes great responsibility", said Peter Parker (Spiderman) and "with freedom comes responsibility" said Eleanor Roosevelt. They were right. Fletcherising is a very powerful tool and it gives immense freedom from diet and exercising restrictions. This does not mean however that, we throw away all our "being nice to ourselves" way of life and go on a comfort food Fletcherising spree. I did that initially, but since Fletcherising eventually teaches you to be responsible, I stabilized as it were. I did feel discouraged though when I realized what I was doing and the impact it would have on my goals. Fortunately it was not very late. It's good to avoid the temptation to suddenly throw away the lifestyle and the food habits you have and let the transition happen naturally. You don't have to force any food on yourself but yes there will be a transition towards food that is completely chewable, which leaves out meat somehow. So yes you may discover that your liking for meat and any such food which leaves remains have diminished. The preferred food will get more and more simple. But again it will be a natural transition and not a forced giving up or depriving, so you don't have to think about it.

Constipation

On this Fletcher says that, "*To illustrate the prevailing ignorance relative to this most important necessity of self care, and also a traditional prejudice, even among physicians, the following extract from a letter just received is given : You ask me to define more exactly what I mean by constipation; this is not at all difficult; I mean skipping a day in having a call to stool. There was no trouble about it, and the quantity was not large, but when I mentioned it to my doctor he advised me to stop chewing if it interfered with the regular daily stools. I must confess that I never felt so well as while I was chewing and sipping, instead of the hasty bolting and gulping which one is apt to do on thoughtless or busy occasions, but I don't think it is worthwhile for a chap to monkey with his hygienic department when he is employing a professional regularly to tell him the latest kink about health*"

There are many of us who suffer from this disease called constipation in our body. Which by the way is the direct result of incorrect eating. Many rely on the fibrous drinks available in the market which keep the bowel movements smoother. This is definitely better than having a constipated and therefore quite uncomfortable feeling in our body.

Come to think of it, we shouldn't be required to take any external supplement to keep any function of the body working. Natures design should take care of it. However because of our conscious / unconscious intervention in Natures plans, we render useless one or the other of the obvious and default settings. Fletcherising helps restore the functioning back to normalcy.

However in the meantime when this transition is taking place, we may need to keep helping ourselves with the supplements we are already using or try and switch to some natural supplements such as warm water where the constipation problem is not in its chronic state.

Once we start Fletcherising the change in the way we feel about our body is fairly and quickly visible. That bloated feeling in the stomach disappears or at least tones down to a great extent. However since our colon is infested with a lot of toxic wastes accumulated since birth, it may take some time to shred this away and hence the need to continue with any of the supplements we may already be taking.

Fletcherising puts a limit on the volume of waste generated and so the urge to eliminate waste may not be very apparent, quick or frequent initially as it used to be. This may be a cause of worry for some. Hence again it is advisable to continue with any of the supplements one is used to taking and then experiment with skipping it once in a week or so.

For me, fortunately, I found my way to Fletcherising before bowel related problems reached serious proportions. Eventually I am sure these little problems that I have accumulated will disappear. However in the interim I support myself with warm water every morning, as much as I can drink and would recommend this to anyone who has the slightest of the problems in this area.

Digestion Ash

There are some conflicting views where it comes to the quantity, quality and frequency of the digestion ash eliminated. With Fletcherising, the quantity eliminated will be bare minimum and very much lower than the quantity of food consumed. There are conflicting views with regard to the color, form, the composition of the waste eliminated. Several health enthusiasts have views sometimes completely in contrast to that of Fletchers experiments and observations in this regard. Some health journals / websites say the outgo has to be equal to the inflow while Fletcher says, it will be very much low in proportion. One logical conclusion that can be derived is that if outgo is to be equal to intake, what's the point where's the nutrition getting absorbed in the body? It therefore seems obvious that if intake is 100, outgo has to be less than 100 because the delta is getting absorbed by the body in the form of nutrition. However rest of the perceptions with regard to the quality and frequency does get confusing and was confusing for me. I spent some time thinking about this and analyzing the data till I kind of understood that digestion ash and other waste produced by our body is the effect of what we consciously process, if we are processing it right that is Fletcherising, the effects will align themselves, sooner than later. If there is no garbage in, there will be no garbage out, is the logical conclusion I arrived at. So yes the quantity eliminated will be much lower for sure but I have stopped paying attention to this area and recommend you too do the same. Let Nature carry out its processes without a constant and keen observer keeping a watch on everything. Let your own experience be your guide with regard to rest of the aspects. Keep the faith and carry on with the good work you have started, Nature will and does take care of the rest.

The urgency of eating

Many of us don't really know what true hunger is, the pleasant anticipatory feeling mentioned earlier. So there is this urgency to eat whenever we feel the "desperate hunger" and when we are desperately hungry we are not in the state of mind to patiently Fletcherise. The aim is to fill up the emptiness developing in the stomach. Sometimes there is not even this hunger, there is just a need to eat, boredom, anger, depression, sadness, stress, all these lower vibrating emotions call for food sometimes. This is emotional eating. This too comes with a desperate need to eat. There is therefore this most important need to get rid of the urgency. Food releases a kind of "high" chemicals, thereby neutralizing the bad mood, but not neutralizing the bad health ensuing because of this emotional eating.

I have been through this emotional eating, greedy eating, and "I've never ever seen food in my life" sort of eating. It was with some difficulty that I could wait my turn to take food at a lunch buffets previously. I was addicted to eating. Nothing I did seemed to help in getting rid of this urgency, this addiction, rather I don't think I tried much to get rid of this addiction. Fletcherising helped me, it will help you! If you just work on making it a habit as noted hereinabove, the urgency will die down eventually and make room for patient, enjoyable experience of Fletcherising

9

The Most Precious Gift to Our Children

In the New Glutton or Epicure, Fletcher narrates the impact of "incorrect eating" on a child's growth, "*An infant was not progressing as it should and failed to gain normally in weight. It was under the charge of a nurse and was being carefully watched. A certain quantity of milk was prescribed for daily nourishment, at prescribed times, in a prescribed manner; but the child did not increase in weight and was "doing poorly." For some reason the nurse was changed and instructions were repeated by the old to the new nurse. In the course of a week the little patient showed signs of marked improvement, both in gain of weight and in general condition. In order to record the particulars of the change the physician questioned the nurse and learned that only one half the nourishment originally prescribed had been given, the new nurse having forgotten or misunderstood the orders.*

The reason the little fellow had been "doing so poorly" under the original prescription was because he had been using up his puny strength getting rid of the excess of food that had been forced upon his little stomach and intestines. When the excess was stopped, so that his digestive apparatus could occupy itself with his real needs, the babe had a surplus of energy for growth and thrived as a rightly nourished child should"

It seems very difficult I understand to teach a child the meaning of will power, focus, economy, strength and endurance etc. but it's not difficult to let them remain Fletcherites. Yes they don't have to be taught to Fletcherise, they are born Fletcherites, every child is a born

Fletcherite. That's the training they receive from our Creator right from the womb, we don't have to do anything to teach them "right eating", they know. All we need to do is get out of the way where it comes to "re-training them to eat."

The fact that babies are born without teeth is a sort of practical demonstration by the Creator, to the baby and to the parents, of the state in which food is supposed to be when it falls down the throat–liquid state. The sucking action of a newborn is designed to excite secretion of Saliva. When you put a tiny little piece of food in a baby's mouth, the salivary glands secrete saliva profusely. Till we force them to speed up, they do eat slow, keeping the food in the mouth for a very long time. They know how to eat, just that some of us parents have actually forgotten how to and think our way is the right way. Children Fletcherise! Just that we change their habits by asking them to finish up quickly so that they don't get late for the school or we don't get late for work. Children learn more by experience, looking up to the grownups, than by being told what to do. If we tell them to chew 32 times and we ourselves don't, they know it's okay not to, we on top of it tell them to hurry up. That's what they do then, they hurry up and carry forward this incorrect eating habit into their teenage, adult life and old age. Their life could become infested with diseases and discomforts of all sorts majorly because we parents unconsciously re-train them in their eating habits.

To me, forcing a child to eat is doing more harm to the child than benefit. It could be a far better option to let the decision be on the child. Of course there are times when the child is sick and may need some forced feeding but apart from these days, let the child decide whether or not to eat at any given point of time.

I have seen parents getting the children hooked to the TV sets so that they can get some time of respite for themselves. They do everything, send their children to school, buy them books and toys, take them to a hundred classes swimming, dance, music, martial arts and what not. The children now a days seem busier than the grownups. All these external needs are taken care of and we believe that in the process, we are contributing to the all round over all development of the child.

These things do help, but what if you could give a more precious gift, the gift of health to your child. It can be given by letting them retain their natural eating habits. This would be far better than all the other good things we keep doing for them.

Spiritual coaching of children could be a tough job for some parents and so they might need some external help. But Fletcherising, is a very physical lesson, a lesson the children have already learnt while in the womb. And if this is going to give them a benefit of health, strength, endurance, responsibility, power, long life, economy and increased will power, helping them retain and groom this habit specially when they develop teeth, would be a priceless gift to our children!

Last but not the Least

Once you start forming this "good" eating habit that is Fletcherising, the life ward movement of your body and mind becomes unstoppable, rather you go singing, dancing, delighted and excited enroute. You will be magically attracted to the perfect food your body needs. Since healthy body cannot be passive, you will automatically be inspired to be active, so an "inspired action of a healthy body" it will be and not a "compulsory exercising to remain healthy".

"Mission Fletcherism" has to be embarked upon with the aim of achieving radiant health, strength and endurance, not just weight loss. Aiming for weight loss is like setting up a sugar factory for molasses which is only the byproduct of sugar–the sugar of heath and well being–the molasses i.e. weight loss is a byproduct.

If there is something that promises good, positive outcomes, a solution to my problems and with no risk whatsoever, no investment of any extra money or any of my resources, no "catch" as it were of any sort or form, rather something which can change my life or saves me some money to say the least, I would consider it profitable to believe in. This is because I am looking for a solution to my problems. That's what I did, I believed in what Fletcherism promised and now my belief holds true!

For me and for most, any help, any solution to our problems, in any shape or form are all acceptable, "all donations accepted". This openness helps in ways our limited thinking's do now allow us to imagine. With Fletcherism, what's there to lose except for some unwanted fat, weight and ill health!

It's okay if you are on a diet, on a salad only diet or a liquid only diet. It's okay if health is not your focus for now, it's okay if there are other important things that you would like to give your time to. It's okay if you want to go with the pills and supplements that promise quick and easy weight loss without any effort whatsoever on your part. Try all of this, as much as you want to, but eventually you would want to come home to yourself, to Nature, to the creator and her ways.

Life is joyous ride, a celebration! Enjoy the ride to the fullest, and celebrate as much as you can. *"You have plenty of good things laid up for many years. Take life easy;* ***Eat, drink and be merry****.",* says Luke 12:19 but ***"Just remember to Fletcherise"****,* says Nature!

Happy Eating, Happy Fletcherising!

www.ingramcontent.com/pod-product-compliance
Lightning Source LLC
Chambersburg PA
CBHW030400290526
45785CB00004B/1844